Physical Environments and Aging: Critical Contributions of M. Powell Lawton to Theory and Practice

Physical Environments and Aging: Critical Contributions of M. Powell Lawton to Theory and Practice has been co-published simultaneously as *Journal of Housing for the Elderly*, Volume 17, Numbers 1/2 2003.

Physical Environments and Aging: Critical Contributions of M. Powell Lawton to Theory and Practice

Rick J. Scheidt
Paul G. Windley
Editors

Physical Environments and Aging: Critical Contributions of M. Powell Lawton to Theory and Practice has been co-published simultaneously as *Journal of Housing for the Elderly*, Volume 17, Numbers 1/2 2003.

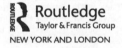

Routledge
Taylor & Francis Group
NEW YORK AND LONDON

First published 2003 by
The Haworth Press, Inc., 10 Alice Street, Binghamton, NY 13904-1580

This edition published 2014 by Routledge
711 Third Avenue, New York, NY 10017
2 Park Square, Milton Park, Abingdon, Oxon OX14 4RN

Routledge is an imprint of the Taylor & Francis Group, an informa business

Physical Environments and Aging: Critical Contributions of M. Powell Lawton to Theory and Practice has been co-published simultaneously as *Journal of Housing for the Elderly*™, Volume 17, Numbers 1/2 2003.

The development, preparation, and publication of this work has been undertaken with great care. However, the publisher, employees, editors, and agents of The Haworth Press and all imprints of The Haworth Press, Inc., including The Haworth Medical Press® and Pharmaceutical Products Press®, are not responsible for any errors contained herein or for consequences that may ensue from use of materials or information contained in this work. Opinions expressed by the author(s) are not necessarily those of The Haworth Press, Inc. With regard to case studies, identities and circumstances of individuals discussed herein have been changed to protect confidentiality. Any resemblance to actual persons, living or dead, is entirely coincidental.

Cover design by Lora Wiggins.

Library of Congress Catalog-in-Publication Data

Physical environments and aging : critical contributions of M. Powell Lawton to theory and practice / Rick J. Scheidt, Paul G. Windley, editors.
    p. ; cm.
"Physical environments and aging : critical contributions of M. Powell Lawton to theory and practice has been co-published simultaneously as Journal of housing for the elderly, Volume 17, Numbers 1/2 2003".
    ISBN 0-7890-2006-8 (alk. Paper) –ISBN 0-7890-2007-6 (pbk : alk. Paper)
    1. Aged–Dwellings–United States. 2. Gerontology. 3. Human beings–Effect of environment on. 4. Environmental psychology. 5. Lawton, M. Powell (Mortimer Powell), 1923- I. Scheidt, Rick J., 1944- II. Windley, Paul G., 1941- III. Journal of housing for the elderly.
    HD7287.92.U54 P49 2003
    362.6–dc21
                                                                                    2002153971

Physical Environments and Aging: Critical Contributions of M. Powell Lawton to Theory and Practice

CONTENTS

ABOUT THE EDITORS

Rick J. Scheidt, PhD, is Professor in the School of Family Studies and Human Services at Kansas State University. His research interests focus on environment-aging relations among older residents of small, rural communities. Most recently, this includes research on deculturation in small, economically-declining ("ghost") towns in Kansas. He is a Fellow of the Gerontological Society of America, the American Psychological Association, and the American Psychological Society. He is a member of the American Association for the Advancement of Science and of the Skeptics Society. He has served on the editorial boards of *The Journal of Gerontology*, *Psychology and Aging*, *Journal of Applied Gerontology*, and *Journal of Housing for the Elderly*. Recent publications include "Successful aging: What's not to like?" (1999), with D. Humpherys and J. Yorgason, *Journal of Applied Gerontology*, 18, 277-282; and "Place therapies for older adults: Conceptual and interventive approaches" (1999), with C. Norris-Baker, *International Journal of Aging and Human Development*, 48, 1-15. He has co-edited the volume *Environment and Aging Theory: A Focus on Housing*, with Paul Windley (1998). He is currently co-editing (with H. W. Wahl and Paul Windley) the *Annual Review of Gerontology and Geriatrics 2003* ("Environments, Gerontology, and Old Age").

Paul G. Windley, D Arch, is Professor of Architecture and past Dean of the College of Art and Architecture at the University of Idaho. He conducts research in environmental gerontology focusing on design and planning issues related to elderly housing and small rural communities. He is a Fellow of the Gerontological Society of America and a member of the Environmental Design Research Association. He was the first Research Associate in Residence with the Herman Miller Research Corporation in Ann Arbor, Michigan, where he conducted research on environmental factors that sustain independent living among older people. Recent publications include: Schmidt, R. J., Windley, P. G. (Eds.), *Environment and Aging Theory: A Focus on Housing*, Greenwood

Press (1998); and *The Maintenance of ADL and IADL Functioning Through Design* (1997), in W. K. Schaie and S. Willis (Eds.), *Societal Mechanisms for Maintaining Competence in Old Age* (Springer Press). He is currently co-editing (with H. W. Wahl and Rick Scheidt) the *Annual Review of Gerontology and Geriatrics 2003* ("Environments, Gerontology, and Old Age").

Introduction

In his beautiful treatise on the many meanings of death, Robert Kastenbaum (1975) discusses the "big death," a death of such significance that it may close one era and open another, "marking a change in how-things-were and how-things-will-be-now" (p. 25). In January of 2001, gerontology suffered such a death with the passing of M. Powell Lawton. In addition to his many definitive contributions to environment-aging studies, Powell Lawton was revered by his friends and colleagues for his steady mentorship and gracious personal support.

In November, 2001, a symposium was offered at the Gerontological Society of America in Chicago to commemorate his work and to pay tribute to his contributions to research, practice, and policy in the realm of the physical environment (widely conceived) and aging. Several of the voices in this volume were part of that original forum. As the GSA presentations ended, the forum was opened to those in the audience who wished to speak about Powell Lawton's influence on their own work. Several attendees came forward and eloquently did so. Benyamin Schwarz, Chief Editor of *Journal of Housing for the Elderly*, graciously invited us (as the symposium organizers) to place these papers–along with those of other invited authors–under one cover, as a tribute to Lawton.

The charge given to the authors was straightforward–to summarize the impact that Lawton's work had on their own fields of inquiry within environment-aging relations. In some instances, the authors of this volume chose to offer clear evaluative summaries of this influence. Others have elected to present original research stimulated by Lawton's tutelage. Many authors insert their personal reflections regarding Lawton the man, as it is difficult to separate his human qualities from the tremendous body of work that marked his professional career. The authors represent at least two distinct cohorts of environment-aging researchers–those that Lawton mentored early on (e.g., Weisman,

[Haworth co-indexing entry note]: "Introduction." Scheidt, Rick J. and Windley, Paul G. Co-published simultaneously in *Journal of Housing for the Elderly* (The Haworth Press, Inc.) Vol. 17, No. 1/2, 2003, pp. 1-4; and: *Physical Environments and Aging: Critical Contributions of M. Powell Lawton to Theory and Practice* (ed: Rick J. Scheidt, and Paul G. Windley) The Haworth Press, Inc., 2003, pp. 1-4. Single or multiple copies of this article are available for a fee from The Haworth Document Delivery Service [1-800-HAWORTH, 9:00 a.m. - 5:00 p.m. (EST). E-mail address: getinfo@haworthpressinc.com].

Regnier, Windley), as well as their students (e.g., Calkins, Chaudhury). The resulting articles form a multi-layered, informative mosaic of his many contributions to the field.

In a contribution that is at once historical and future-directed, Schwarz traces the evolving legacy of Lawton's pervasive influence on research and practice in environment-aging studies. He adopts as a framework for discussion dilemmas inherent in three issues that captured Lawton's attention throughout his prolific career–basic versus applied research; theory-driven versus empirically-directed research and practice; and the discerning of boundaries between persons and environments. Schwarz thoughtfully "unpacks" the meanings of these multi-layered issues in Lawton's work, including their diverse implications for current and future research in environment-aging studies, as well as practice and policy that targets purpose-built housing. It is a fitting introductory framework for this volume, as these prism-like themes are certainly reflected in diverse ways within each of the other contributions.

Weisman and Moore examine Lawton's contributions to the most fundamental assumptions of environment-aging research–the philosophical foundations of the paradigms that guided his thinking and research. These were not trivial or esoteric issues for Lawton. As they note, "Lawton explored a variety of philosophical positions and continued to work toward a meaningful synthesis of what are often seen as conflicting world views." The authors usefully examine the implications of five complementary perspectives–axiological, ontological, epistemological, methodological, and praxeological–for applied research professionals and do a masterful job illustrating the relevance of these issues for environment-aging researchers and practitioners working to improve everyday environments of older adults.

From the other end of the spectrum, Regnier reviews Lawton's contributions to the built-environment, focusing specifically on major principles of design and planning emerging from Lawton's volume, *Planning and Managing Housing for the Elderly* (1975). Specifically, Regnier shares with us 10 critical, discipline-crossing issues that urged a "transactional partnership" between planners and managers, influenced the way other researchers approached environmental design research, and established the foundation for design guidelines and housing manuals for the 1980s. They encompass the role of older individuals themselves as well as the broader community context in providing supportive and optimal built-environments for older adults.

Lawton conducted a considerable amount of his research among community populations at physical, personal, suprapersonal, and social environmental levels (to use his own taxonomy). Scheidt and Norris-Baker offer a selective review of his contributions to work in each of these arenas, including the relevance of the Ecological Theory of Aging for understanding coping among older community residents; seminal work on community planning; the role of emotion as a determinant, moderator, and outcome of environmental adjustment and place attachment; and Lawton's novel use of time as a research dimension. The authors illustrate the multiple meanings that community held for Lawton as a context for successful aging.

Calkins moves us to the context of long-term care facilities, showing how Lawton's work in this arena contributed to the radical design changes that have occurred over the past three decades. She discusses the influence of several of Lawton's key environmental principles for people with dementia–orientation, negotiability, personalization, social interaction, and safety–and nicely illustrates their expression in contemporary (state-of-the-art) long-term care design. It is here, perhaps more clearly than any other application, that Lawton's conceptions of environmental support, security, and optimization blended so tractably to benefit vulnerable elders. Calkins reviews empirical research that supports the validity of this claim.

The intriguing therapeutic possibilities which emerge from the realization that "sense of self" is intrinsically related to "sense of place" are examined by Chaudhury. Specifically, Chaudhury discusses the relevance of Lawton's multidimensional "good life" model for his own developing theory and research on "place therapy." Using both theoretical and exploratory empirical illustrations from his own work, he demonstrates the therapeutic value of autobiographical place-based reminiscence for cognitively-intact elders and those with dementia residing in adult care facilities. Chaudhury discusses future applications of place-oriented recollection that may affect positive outcomes in the quality of life for older adults, particularly those with dementia.

Lawton believed that in order for individuals to successfully age-in-place, residential environments must be changed to accommodate the changes brought about by declines in functional abilities. Pynoos, Nishita, and Perelman discuss Lawton's pioneering contributions to the theory and research on home modification. They review and illustrate how developments in home modification research, assessment approaches, and the service delivery system can be attributed to his influence. Also, they evaluate major problems with home modification programs, discuss existing programs and "best approaches," and share research on their effectiveness.

Lawton was aware early on that the psychological well-being of older adults is greatly impacted by their ability to maintain a sense of control over their immediate physical environment in the face of age-related functional declines, particularly in domains of sensory acuity as well as strength and flexibility. Koncelik traces Lawton's contributions to both research and product design in the micro-environmental human factors sphere. He also discusses the particular responsibility of the designer in addressing issues of safety, security, and sense of satisfaction of elders who must live with the designs produced by others. In his sweeping and useful treatment, Koncelik traces Lawton's influence on the "product environment," reviews usual (normative) functional ability losses so frequently experienced by older adults, their meanings for functioning in the near environment, and how design and product changes in specific functional spaces can enhance adaptation for them. Koncelik's analysis provides a useful micro-level companion to Pynoos' et al. broader view regarding home modification.

Powell Lawton recognized that the most elegant constructs, whether environmental or person-oriented, are only as valid as the measures developed to represent them. He was a meticulous and careful psychometrician who loved the challenge of doing science with the constructs he posed. Therefore, in concert with the previous articles on the significance of control over the household and immediately adjacent environment, it seems fitting that our volume closes with a focus on a new measure of household control. Acknowledging the influence of Lawton on their work, Oswald, Wahl, Martin, and Mollenkopf (of the University of Heidelberg) unveil a new measure–the Housing-Related Control Beliefs Questionnaire (HCQ) assessing Internal Control, External Control: Powerful Others, and External Control: Chance. They present two validation studies, examining the psychometric integrity of the measure in the context of Socio-structural variables, general control beliefs, and objective and subjective housing-related variables. Their findings support the potential usefulness of the HCQ as a measure of environmental proactivity in late adulthood.

Environmental gerontology will certainly not be the same without Powell Lawton. His work spanned all dimensions of good science from theoretical development, to taxonomic development for both behavioral and environmental domains, to methodological innovations, and finally to application for a variety of disciplines represented by articles in this volume. We take heart in the knowledge that he mentored and taught so well, and has left a legacy on which future scholars and researchers can build.

Rick J. Scheidt
Paul G. Windley

REFERENCES

Kastenbaum, R. (1975). Is death a life crisis? On the confrontation with death in theory and practice. In N. Datan & L. Ginsberg (Eds.), *Life-span developmental psychology: Normative life crises* (pp. 19-50). New York: Academic Press.

Lawton, M.P. (1975). *Planning and managing housing for the elderly.* New York: John Wiley and Sons.

M. Powell Lawton's Three Dilemmas in the Field of Environment and Aging

Benyamin Schwarz

SUMMARY. Three scholarly dilemmas have characterized Powell Lawton's career: basic versus applied research; theory-driven versus empirically-dominated research; and the intrinsic psychological dilemma of person-environment transactions. These themes serve as an organizing framework for the analysis of the discipline of environment and aging studies. Researchers in this field share a social mission as well as the responsibility to gain theoretical and applied knowledge for intervention that can improve the quality of older people's lives. At the same time, research in this field hinges on the willingness of those who are supposed to benefit from the research, to try it out, and use the results. The chapter is an attempt to use Lawton's seminal contribution to this field in order to look to the future of theory, practice and policy in environment-aging studies. *[Article copies available for a fee from The Haworth Document Delivery Service: 1-800-HAWORTH. E-mail address: <getinfo@haworthpressinc.com> Website: <http://www.HaworthPress.com> © 2003 by The Haworth Press, Inc. All rights reserved.]*

KEYWORDS. Basic versus applied research, theory, person-environment transaction

---

Benyamin Schwarz is affiliated with the University of Missouri-Columbia.

[Haworth co-indexing entry note]: "M. Powell Lawton's Three Dilemmas in the Field of Environment and Aging." Schwarz, Benyamin. Co-published simultaneously in *Journal of Housing for the Elderly* (The Haworth Press, Inc.) Vol. 17, No. 1/2, 2003, pp. 5-22; and: *Physical Environments and Aging: Critical Contributions of M. Powell Lawton to Theory and Practice* (ed: Rick J. Scheidt, and Paul G. Windley) The Haworth Press, Inc., 2003, pp. 5-22. Single or multiple copies of this article are available for a fee from The Haworth Document Delivery Service [1-800-HAWORTH, 9:00 a.m. - 5:00 p.m. (EST). E-mail address: getinfo@haworthpressinc.com].

Much has been written in recent years–all of it true–about Powell Lawton's unique blend of strength and unpretentious personality, leadership, and unassuming character. He was "always his own man," noted Elaine Brody in her Foreword to *The Many Dimensions of Aging*, "his independence of thinking, soaring intelligence, pristine conceptualizations, meticulous insistence on accuracy, prodigious capacity for work, encyclopedic knowledge, astonishing output, adventurous explorations–one could go on and on without exhausting the inventory of good things that characterize his work" (2000, p. xvii). The editors of the same collection concurred: "His friendly, loyal, and supportive nature has made him mentor and colleague to many. Despite working full-time at a research institution, the Polisher Research Institute of the Philadelphia Geriatric Center, he has mentored dozens, if not hundreds, of students and young scholars and researchers" (Rubinstein et al., 2000, p. xix).

I was attending graduate school at the College of Architecture at the University of Michigan when I first met Powell Lawton. By that time I had read several of his books and articles on environment and aging, which were already considered seminal works in this discipline. To my surprise, rather than speaking on the Ecological Theory of Aging (Lawton & Nahemow, 1973), Lawton focused the discussion on the role of caregivers in long-term care. I remember being amazed by the rigor of Powell's statistical analysis (which I hardly understood), and the depth of his knowledge when he answered the questions from the audience, who represented a wide spectrum of disciplines. When the session ended, I went and introduced myself. I was touched by his sincere curiosity about my background, and his warm encouragement regarding my interest in the architecture of long-term care settings.

Since that time, we met several times in annual meetings of the Gerontological Society of America (GSA) and the Environmental Design Research Association (EDRA). Surrounded by students and well-wishers, Powell always had insightful comments on the presentations, urging us to examine what we'd done–and how to do it better the next time. He felt the glee in other researchers' success–a feeling that only a truly modest person can feel. On one of these occasions, I asked him whether he was the "blind" reviewer of the manuscript of a book I co-edited with my colleague (Schwarz & Brent, 1999). I suspected that he had reviewed the book, because the comments that we received from the publisher were typed on an old typewriter similar to the one he used in our correspondence. Powell smiled kindly in the smile that his friends so loved, and generously admitted that he was the reviewer. We thanked him for his advice and honest critique and asked him to contribute a foreword for the book, which he graciously agreed to write.

* * *

Three scholarly dilemmas have characterized Powell Lawton's career. He listed them in his intellectual autobiography:

> The dilemma of knowledge at the service of the people versus knowledge as a scholarly goal in its own right, or applied versus basic science, was my first dilemma in a chronological sense and perhaps in overall importance. A second source of tension in the practice of research is the degree to which theory directs scientific work versus the degree to which empirical approaches predominate. Third, environmental psychology's intrinsic dilemma is to define what is person and what is environment, or are they? These three dilemmas constitute parallel threads that bind this writer's intellectual career, but to some extent, the order in which they have been named here is both their chronological order and their order of increasing differentiation. (Lawton, 1990: 340)

Contemplating the future of Environment and Aging, this essay will use these three dilemmas as a framework for discussion.

BASIC VERSUS APPLIED RESEARCH

According to his own testimony, Powell entered the evolving field of Gerontology in 1963, when new federal programs for purposely designed housing for older people and age-segregated public housing had just begun to be developed. Prior to the early 1960s most elderly people and their families were ignored, and largely existed as a neglected part of the American society. Old people were poor, economically dependent on their children. The Older Americans Act did not exist yet, and Supplemental Security Income was established almost 10 years later. Medicare and Medicaid were still being deliberated in Congress, and when the Social Security Act Amendment finally passed in 1965, it radically transformed the delivery of medical care in the U.S. At the time the new law was implemented there was virtually no specialized housing for the elderly, nor long-term care services. The majority of the nation's nursing homes were unable to meet Medicare standards for extended-care facilities, and some homes were even having difficulties meeting Medicaid's loose, interim skilled nursing home regulations.

Increasing numbers of older people in need of housing and services, the establishment of new forms of housing arrangements for the elderly, and the linkage of the two phenomena through applied research helped to launch the field of Environment and Aging.

Chronologically earlier and totally consistent with the applied thrust of the research, an atheoretical empirical approach to housing research was extraordinarily well-suited to produce information that could be consumed by a waiting audience. Planners wanted to know the kinds of services potential clients would want. Administrators wanted to know how satisfied clients were with different design features. Architects wanted to know what features would be used most frequently or what would be associated with better outcomes. Theses applied issues addressed in this research demanded a head-counting, empirical approach, but its results led to the docility hypothesis, a theoretically relevant contribution. (Lawton, 1990: 346)

Thus, the demand for applied research and the wish to improve the lives of the growing number of elderly people propelled Environmental Gerontology in these formative years. First there was relevant, applied research. Theory development came later, with the common scientific knowledge that applied research could be improved when driven by theoretically meaningful concepts. Congressional committees, the Department of Housing and Urban Development, the Administration on Aging, the Farmers Home Administration, and even the White House were genuinely interested in studies about environment and aging during the 1970s and the early 1980s. These agencies and many other organizations funded research, facilitated the dissemination of research findings, and influenced "such areas as the national policy in congregate housing, design standards for housing, and the design of institutions" (Lawton, 1990: 347).

We are living in different times. While housing accommodations and services options for older people developed beyond recognition over the last several decades, interest in environment and aging research as well as funding opportunities for this line of inquiry, have noticeably eroded. Complex economic, political, and sociological pressures brought about the lack of attention and financial support from the service-providing sector and the policy making sector. Regrettably, discussion of this disturbing situation is beyond the scope of this essay. A brief quote will suffice:

Several factors may be responsible for the lull in empirical research during the past decades. One possible explanation is the relative standstill in federally assisted housing program development since 1980. Similar factors are the relatively small trickle of new nursing home construction and the slowing of community development funds, both of which spurred the research in the 1970s. Another trend that resulted at least partly from diminished federal funds was the somewhat belated interest of the policy and housing services professions in older persons living in ordinary communities. (Parmelee & Lawton, 1990: 464)

Research is dependent on those who nourish it materially and provide time, space and money to produce it. Research is "ultimately the fruit of the social and political world that shares enough beliefs and values with those who do the research to allow them to do so, to accept the risk of their failures and claim some credit for their successes" (Habraken, 1979: 4). Researchers in the field of environment and aging share a social mission as well as the responsibility to gain theoretical and applied knowledge for intervention that can improve the quality of older people's lives. At the same time, research in this field hinges on the willingness of those who are supposed to benefit from the research, to try it out, and use the results. The definitive test of the "success" of any research results lies in the question of whether those results will be accepted or rejected by the social body that they are supposed to benefit.

Like many other researchers in the field, I believe that "theory is practice, and must stand and fall with its practicality, provided that the mode and contexts of its applications be suitably specified" (Kaplan, 1964). If a design theory for creating better environments for frail elderly people, for example, "is not helpful in making design decisions leading to predictable outcomes, then it is irrelevant" (Lang, 1987). To remain relevant, we have to ensure that our studies not only determine causal relationships among variables with the hope of producing significant results, but we also need to generate knowledge sufficiently meaningful to affect elderly people, their families, providers of care, and policy makers.

In a perfect world, "basic and applied aspects merge and mutually reinforce one another" (Lawton, 1990: 349). In reality, however, basic and applied research differ in purpose, context and methods. While applied research strives to improve life and solve real-life problems, basic research is not intended to solve problems, or at least this is not its motivating force. The basic researcher is usually investigating narrowly focused questions, which enable him or her to concentrate on a single measurement task in a relatively controlled environment. In contrast, the applied researcher tends to perform his or her investigation in an uncontrolled environment, facing multiple ill-constrained, ill-framed questions that often come from the client (Hedric, Bickman, & Rog, 1993). Even when the questions are well defined, the environment is a complex one and can impose special demands on the applied researcher.

Contemplating on the dilemma of basic versus applied research, Lawton proposed two strategies for researchers in the field of person-environment:

> The first is post-hoc basic research, where research is formulated to answer a question relevant to a social need but the design is determined in such a way as to add to the knowledge base in a form generalizable beyond the present social need. (1990: 350)

Examples of studies that combine basic and applied research are some of the well-known studies that Lawton himself conducted in housing for older people (1976). In a more recent example, Steven Golant (1998) outlined a conceptual model designed to explain personal and environmental outcomes experienced by elders following changes in their shelter and care setting. Emphasizing a temporal perspective that recognizes the individuality of each person in a new setting and the congruence of this setting with the person's needs, the model attempts to go beyond models that have dealt with the consequences of older people's moves into various residential settings. Golant rightly warns against homogenizing groups of older people "simply because they currently are attributed with having identical characteristics or experiences" (p. 36). Intended both for analytical and practical applications, the model delineates a complex construct of particular characteristics that direct elders' assessment of their care setting.

The second strategy Lawton proposed is aimed at the environment in the Person-Environment dichotomy. As he noted:

> The second practice-directed research strategy is simple design-problem research done to provide guidance to those responsible for decisions regarding the person-made environment. (1990: 351)

Studies in this vein include Zeisel, Epp, and Demos (1978); Zeisel, Welch, Epp, and Demos (1983); Howell (1980); Cohen and Weisman (1991); Cohen and Day (1993); Hoglund and Ledewitz (1999); Regnier, Hamilton, and Yatabe (1995); and Lemke and Moos (2001). These examples of applied research can be attributed to the recognition that the physical environment has a significant, perhaps central, role in enhancing therapeutic processes. However, Lawton cautioned us about the "wicked nature of the relationship between basic knowledge and practice." He noted that:

> Synthesis is rarely a feasible goal in reaching an informed design solution because the demand for practical solutions always outstrips the resources of basic science to deliver them. Thus the researcher faces the dilemma of communicating unsatisfying small amounts of knowledge derived from research that meets acceptable methodological standards or, on the other hand, going significantly beyond the data so as to provide concrete design assistance. Either way someone loses, the practitioner in frustration over the limited amount of guidance available from the academic, or the researcher in risking a loss of integrity in going beyond the data. (Lawton, 1990: 351)

The dilemma of basic versus applied research can be traced all the way to Immanuel Kant (1724-1804), who "revived a distinction, found in Aristotle, between theoretical and practical knowledge. *Theoretical knowledge* refers to states of affairs whose existence can be checked, tested and accepted. *Practical knowledge*, on the other hand, refers to decision making" (Hamilton, 1994: 63). Thus we may look again at Powell Lawton's work, which had always been linked to the application of theoretical knowledge through moral judgments and interventions in the domain of environment for older people. He taught us that in the realm of environment and aging, applied research is about social justice, and that "what to do relates not only to what is, but also to inseparable notions of what ought to be" (Hamilton, 1994: 63).

THEORETICAL VERSUS EMPIRICAL RESEARCH

To begin the discussion of the second dilemma Lawton explored in his intellectual autobiography, we may need first to talk about the meaning of theory and empirical research. *The Oxford English Dictionary* defines theory as a "scheme or system of ideas or statements held as an explanation or account of a group of facts or phenomena; a hypothesis that has been confirmed or established by observation or experiment, and is propounded or accepted as accounting for the known facts; a statement of what are held to be general laws, principles, or causes of something known or observed." Some of the characteristics of a theory, not found in this definition, include its explanatory and predictive power, and its ability to derive a myriad of descriptive statements from a single explanatory assertion.

When Lawton acknowledged "the power of good theory to direct basic research and ultimately practice" (1990: 353), he pointed out one of the roles of scientific theory, which is to provide the dynamic and rationale of science, as well as to be the source of its universality. In this context, "theories tell us where to look, what to look for, and what to make of what we see" (Rouse, 1987: 100). The triumph of science as the most successful means we have devised to date for constructing and improving representations of the world has been traditionally attributed to empiricism. Empirical research focuses on testing of theoretical representations "against carefully controlled observation and reporting of relevant features of the world, followed by the revision or replacement of those theories that fail to correspond to what is observed" (Rouse, 1987: 3).

Immanuel Kant defined knowledge independent of experience and all impressions of the senses as a priori knowledge, and distinguished it from empirical knowledge, which has its sources a posteriori, that is, in experience. Lawton

(1990) used the term empirics in a different connotation. He emphasized the importance of atheoretical research in environment and behavior and attempted to show the importance of data collection from existing, yet neglected sources. Concerned about the future of his field of research, Lawton discussed the contribution of descriptive data and post-occupancy evaluations to scientific knowledge:

> Most fields recognize better than do psychology the necessity for defining the usual as a beginning point for understanding variability and deviation. Perhaps because description is the first phase of developing a science, there is a compulsion to prove one's sophistication by moving quickly beyond description toward explanation and control. Neither botany nor chemistry would ever have gone far, however, without the Linnaean classification or the periodic table. (1990: 353-354)

This section focuses on the relationships between scientific, theoretical and empirical research as opposed to the theoretical versus atheoretical research that was discussed by Lawton in his autobiography.

It was Thomas Kuhn, in his seminal text *The Structure of Scientific Revolutions*, who first invoked the notion of a *paradigm* to explain the practice of science. Kuhn used the concept in two distinct meanings: *disciplinary matrix*, and exemplar. Kuhn's first usage of the term paradigm is as a *global theory* that embodies the fundamental theories and concepts accepted at a particular time in a field of research. Accordingly, a disciplinary matrix is "the entire constellation of beliefs, values, techniques and so on shared by members of a given community" (Kuhn, 1970: 175). This set of theoretical doctrines constituting a worldview serves several functions for the researchers who engage in this line of inquiry:

> It prescribes some beliefs as essential and proscribes others. It determines which facts it is important to know and provides some general expectations of what those facts will be. These expectations will not always be met, however. Such failures or anomalies, provide the puzzles that keep normal science occupied. Normal science is essentially puzzle solving, attempting to reduce the discrepancies between a paradigmatic worldview and the world and to fill in the many blanks left open by the original sketchy development of the worldview. The distinctive feature of such puzzle solving is that it cannot challenge the fundamental beliefs taken from the paradigm. If a scientist fails to reconcile theory and evidence, it represents a failure of the scientist, not the theory. A paradigm guides puzzle solving in three ways: its values determine which puzzles are worth solving and what those solutions are supposed to achieve; the paradigm specifies the standards for acceptable solutions to puzzles; and

finally, paradigms suggest model problem solutions (exemplars) that heuristically guide scientists toward such solutions. (Rouse, 1987: 27-28)

While many philosophers of science paid attention to the use of the term paradigm as a *global theory*, Kuhn's second mode of usage of the term as an *exemplar* is the one that he "himself saw as central in understanding how scientists learn to make sense of the world through finding ways of bridging indeterminacies and making judgments in conditions of uncertainty" (Turnbull, 2000: 8). Kuhn's usage of paradigm as *exemplar* suggests that "paradigms are not primarily agreed-upon theoretical commitments but exemplary ways of conceptualizing and intervening in particular empirical contexts. Accepting a paradigm is more like acquiring and applying a skill than like understanding and believing a statement" (Rouse, 1987: 30). Furthermore, exemplars are products of tacit knowledge, which is "learned by doing science rather than by acquiring rules for doing it" (Kuhn, 1970: 191).

Perhaps the only model in the field of environment and aging that deserves to be called a paradigm, or an *exemplar* based on Kuhn's second definition of the term, is Lawton and Nahemow's *Adaptation Model* (1973). The model, which was labeled also as the *Ecological Model of Environment and Aging* or *The Ecological Theory of Aging* (Nahemow, 2000), has been described in several publications including this collection (see Weisman & Diaz-Moore), and is recognized as one of the most "prominent middle-range theories" in the field. The model takes into account an individual's competence to cope with environmental press and views the problem of functioning as one matching an individual's fitness for the most appropriate setting. The central concept of the theory is the adaptation level, which mediates between the individual's competence and the environmental press. The theory generally proposes that people "who operate at higher levels of competence can adapt to a wider range of environmental press and have greater likelihood of experiencing favorable adaptive outcomes. Those of lower competence will experience a greater range of press in negative terms, exhibiting a narrower range of adaptive behavior" (Scheidt & Windley, 1985: 248).

Powell Lawton spent a significant part of his professional life furthering this model. However, despite several decades of using the model in different ways, theoreticians in the field of environment and aging have been disturbed by the fact that the theory has not been sufficiently tested. For instance, Scheidt and Windley (1985) claim that Lawton (1982) cited numerous examples of studies supporting the principles of the ecological model; however, despite the generalization of the model, they criticize, little research "has been conducted with the intent of directly testing the formal relations of the model" (p. 248). More recently, Lucille Nahemow (2000), who developed the model with Powell

Lawton, listed numerous studies that tested the model, generated hypotheses from it, used it as a basis for environmental assessment, employed it as a springboard for new models and utilized it as a political tool. She maintained, however, that "clearly, much more research is needed to test the theory; unfortunately prospective, well-controlled studies are expensive and rare. It has been much more common for researchers to use the [Ecological Theory of Aging] to generate research hypotheses" (p. 27).

Testing theories is important because it enables researchers to refine or correct them. Scientists treat science as a construction and appraisal of theories, which intend to represent the world. They construct models that represent certain phenomena in the world, and then using other models and theories, they observe what happens in various situations to test whether their models and theories can portray things accurately. "The discrepancies that show up, and the new phenomena that appear, lead to the construction of new theories or models that are themselves tested in the same way, and so on" (Rouse, 1987: 39).

To paraphrase Ian Hacking (1983), we may stress the significance of testing theories because it often takes its own course, exploring areas not yet theoretically articulated. This is where theoretical and empirical research come together. Testing theories "does more than fill in the gaps left by prior theorizing or check its adequacy. It opens new domains for investigation, refines them to make them suitable for theoretical reflection, and provides a practical grasp of that domain as a resource" (Rouse, 1987: 100-101).

Scholars in the field of environment and aging frequently raise the question of whether the field needs to converge on a paradigm, or whether it can remain in a state of constant flux. At the end of his book, Kuhn (1970) implies that in some fields, scientists are unwilling to commit themselves to a single paradigm. It is argued that the strength as well as the weakness of the environment and aging field stem from its multidisciplinarity. While interdisciplinary research can benefit the field, diversity leads frequently to a lack of overlap between the interest and work of the design-oriented and the social-oriented researchers (Lawton, 1990a). Due to this diversity, I suspect that the field of environment and aging will never adhere for long to a single paradigm because researchers in this line of inquiry address distinct, sometimes opposite questions for which no paradigm will suffice. The field will continue to be eclectic, pluralistic, and syncretic. And researchers will go on to pursue "their theoretical assumptions and working practices from a marketplace of ideas" (Hamilton, 1994: 61).

As for the dilemma of theoretical versus empirical research, Abraham Kaplan echoed the same quandaries when he observed:

In the conduct of inquiry we are continuously subjected to pulls in opposite directions: to search for data or to formulate hypotheses, to construct theories or to perform experiments, to focus on general laws or on individual cases, to conduct molar studies or molecular ones, to engage in synthesis or in analysis. It is seldom of much help, in the concrete, to be told that we must do both. (1964: 40)

Through his lifelong work Powell Lawton taught us that when we face these quandaries, we cannot make a choice of the lesser of two evils and put up with the disappointing outcomes. The problems that these dilemmas pose cannot be solved, but only coped with. One just hopes to learn to live with these dilemmas with the same poise with which Lawton dealt with them.

PERSON VERSUS ENVIRONMENT

Ittelson (1973), who was quoted by Lawton (1990) as being one of the greatest minds in this field, observed:

The environment involves the active participation of all aspects. Man is never concretely encountered independent of the situation through which he acts, nor is the environment ever encountered independent of the encountering individual. It is meaningless to speak of either as existing apart from the situation in which it is encountered. The word "transaction" has been used to label such a situation, for the word carries a double implication: One, all parts of the situation enter into it as active participants: and two, these parts owe their very existence as encountered in a situation to such active participation–they do not appear as already existing entities which merely interact with each other without affecting their own identity. (pp. 18-19)

Altman and Rogoff's (1987) transactional perspective of was adopted by Parmelee and Lawton (1990) as a better representation of the person-environment (P-E) process. According to this approach people and their environment are an inseparable entity. "The transactional model further stresses the dynamic, changing quality of P-E relations rather than static characteristics of individuals and their physical world" (p. 477). The interactional approach to the relationships between older persons' behavior and the environment introduced the subject-object problem into the philosophical foundation of environment and aging studies. This dualistic concept of the individual allowed two simultaneous but mutually exclusive interpretations under which the theories of environmental gerontology would be developed. At the same time it created a fundamental problem: On the one hand, the older individual is perceived as one of "the elderly," whose actions and behavior are determined by the external forces of the environment; on the other hand, the individual is seen as a freely thinking, freely acting subject whose actions and behavior are determined by his or her own personal inner drives and desires. The problems that emerge from this duality revolve around two issues: Is the individual's behavior determined by conditions in his or her environment, or in his or her own internal wiring? and How can the environment and the person interactively shape each other?

Lawton acknowledged that the multiple layering of person-environment transaction has made the use of the qualitative mode of data collection and analysis the most appropriate method for the study of transaction. He used qualitative observations and interviews in an environmental research he described (Lawton, 1985). A team consisting of a social worker, an architect, a psychologist, and an occupational therapist conducted a research project in 50 homes of impaired older people. The purpose of the study was "to learn about deficiencies in the physical quality of the home and the way people coped with them" (Lawton, 1990, p. 357). Besides the use of qualitative observations and personal interviews, the research demonstrated the benefit of multidisciplinarity. Gerontology began as a multidisciplinary endeavor; however, little research in this discipline to date truly lives up to the definition of interdisciplinarity (Achenbaum, 1995). The study Lawton and his colleagues conducted attests to the fact that research in environment and aging can benefit from more multidisciplinary investigations and collaborations among scholars who dare to cross the borders of their respective disciplines and conduct research that can yield practical outcomes for elderly people.

The choice of research methods in the study of the several levels of complexity in person-environment relations depends on many factors; however, Parmelee and Lawton (1990) argued that the more complex levels "require more global concepts and that, for the present, qualitative approaches to empirical research are better able to deal with such concepts" (p. 477).

Accordingly, Robert Rubinstein (1998) traced the origin of the theoretical foundations of the phenomenology of housing for elderly people. He focused on the individual and cultural experience of older persons concerning their dwellings in order to enrich our understanding of the meaning of place in old age. Rubinstein's phenomenological approach to the interrelationship of person and home complements the conventional assumptions of scholars in the area of environment and aging, who have tended to ignore sociocultural, psychological and experiential aspects "in the context of the life course associations of person and place" (p. 93). Rubinstein discussed theories concerning the home as an experiential phenomenon for older adults, the concept of aging in place, the process of place attachment, and the phenomenology of home habituation as these are embedded in the larger social circumstances. Rubinstein's use of ethnographic approaches and qualitative methods to improve our understanding of person-environment relationships corresponds with the views of other experts on aging, trained in the humanities, who in recent years "have begun to subvert the assumption that gerontology should be classified primarily as a 'science' " (Achenbaum, 1995: 253).

The introduction of qualitative methods to the study of transaction between person and environment highlights the alleged differences between the philosophies of qualitative and quantitative methods. Both methods have their relative strengths and weaknesses. Some of these differences are synonymous with the distinctions between the natural sciences and the human sciences. The following is a partial list based on Rouse (1987):

1. Data in natural sciences are usually indisputable. They are identical to any observer. The human sciences, on the other hand, "deal with meaningful objects and situations, whose interpretation is always potentially open to challenge based upon different interpreter's interests, situations, or prior beliefs" (p. 46).
2. While theories in natural sciences are explanatory constructs, the human sciences strive for understanding, not explanation.
3. "Natural scientific theories are either confirmed or falsified by data that can be identified and described without reference to theory" (p. 46). In human sciences the collected information is revealed through some kind of interpretation.
4. "The natural sciences aim to eliminate anthropocentric reference or connotations from their concepts, whereas the human sciences inevitably refer to human being's interests, goals, beliefs, and feelings" (p. 46).
5. While natural sciences strive for universal knowledge, the human sciences aim also for local knowledge.

Patton (1990) lists several characteristics of qualitative and quantitative methods. "Qualitative methods permit the evaluator to study selected issues in depth and detail" (p. 13). Quantitative methods "require the use of standardized measures so that the varying perspectives and experiences of people can be fit into a limited number of predetermined response categories, to which numbers are assigned" (p. 14). The small sample size of qualitative studies often limits the possibilities of generalization. There are deeper philosophical issues involved in this limitation. Patton (1990) distinguished between scientists–a quantitative researcher and evaluators–a qualitative investigator. He noted:

> While scientists search for universal laws and generalizations across time and space, evaluators tend to focus on providing useful information

that is fairly specific to one or a few programs. Moreover, qualitative evaluators tend to be philosophically and methodologically skeptical of generalizations based on statistical inferences drawn from data collected at one or a few points in a program's life. Findings based on samples, however large, are often stripped of their context when generalizations are made–particularly generalizations across time and space. (pp. 486-487)

While validity in quantitative research depends on the measuring instrument and its adequate administration, "in qualitative inquiry the researcher is the instrument" (Patton, 1990: 14). Therefore, the validity in this mode of inquiry depends on the skill, proficiency, and rigor of the researcher in the field.

Despite the limitation of the qualitative mode, Lawton argued that qualitative observations and conceptual creativity led the concept of transactionalism toward theory development. He noted:

This approach has fed every stream of application in the design professions because the levels of generality of transactional concepts are the same level of art practiced by planners and architects as they strive to operationalize means toward the achievement of human goals–that is, highly generalized and conceptual. (1990: 359)

At the same time Parmelee and Lawton (1990) acknowledged the need for longitudinal studies, which mix qualitative and quantitative methods to measure person and environment transaction. They argued that this combination "offers the best opportunity to move the field beyond its current languishing state" (p. 483). Scholars in environmental gerontology have generally shared this view but the progress in theoretical research on the transactional aspects of person-environment has been limited (Wahl, 2001). Lawton himself agreed that:

the transactional aspects may be the most difficult of all to measure. These aspects include the ways in which–and the extent to which–the environment affects interpersonal processes such as cognition; affect; motivation; behavior in relation to the external environment; impacts of this behavior on the environment; and feedback of the changed environment to another cycle of person-environment (P-E) transaction. (1990a: 289)

While researchers in the field of environment and aging continue to study the multiple competences and other characteristics of the person, environmental attributes have not been studied in same pace, as Lawton (1998) stated: "Advances in environmental knowledge have not been matched by advances in knowledge regarding the person and individual differences in the person-environment transaction" (Lawton, 1998: 2). One of Lawton's aspirations centered on improving the taxonomy of the environment:

> The environment has yet to be subjected to a successful classificatory effort. If we knew the most meaningful dimensions of the environment and how they were related to one another, this taxonomy would be enormously useful in the further development of the science of person/environment relations, much as the periodic table served this function in chemistry. (Lawton, 1980: 17)

Similar ambition was echoed in Lawton's later work (Lawton, 1999) and in the *Environmental Design Lexicon for Dementia Care* project that Lawton initiated and never had the opportunity to conclude. However, the complexity of the environmental context has made the task of compiling taxonomies very problematical and, perhaps even counterproductive. The difficulty evidently derives from the multilayered character of the physical, social, psychological, and behavioral elements of the environment. These often produce inconclusive debates and disciplinary discords rather than harmony.

Lawton believed that the research on the environmental aspect of the person-environment transaction can gain significantly from the collaboration among design professionals and scientists, as he proposed: "It is possible that a deliberate attempt to fortify the multidisciplinary character of future research teams will provide the empirical research with a better supply of creative and design-relevant ideas" (1990a: 303-304). The collaboration of designers and researchers in environmental gerontology is important because any attempt by researchers to test what they do, how it influences their potential users, or how it can be changed has to be done in conjunction with environmental designers. As Habraken explained: "Any formulation of a design theory is an attempt to describe the behavior of designers. Any introduction of a design method is, finally, an attempt to change the behavior of people who design. Research in design is therefore doubly connected to the social fabric" (1979: 5).

To study the physical environment on the theoretical level we need to understand the role of theory in architecture. In this sense we need to distinguish between positive or analytic theories and normative theories (Lang, 1987). Scientific theories are analytic, rational constructs intended to understand the principles of how the world is, while some of the architectural theories are normative guidelines that are telling us how the world should be. Hillier (1996) clarified the need for the two kinds of theories in architecture:

> Theories in science are set of general, abstract ideas through which we understand and interpret the material phenomena the world offers to our experience. They deal with how the world is, not how it might be. Be-

cause architecture is creative it requires theories of possibility in the sense that they exist in art. But because architecture is also predictive, it needs analytic theories of actuality as well as theories of possibility. It is this double nature that makes architectural theories unique. They require at once to have the generative power of theories in art and at the same time the analytic power of theories in science. (p. 64)

Therefore the taxonomy of the environment that Lawton had dreamed about was perhaps the first step for a wealth of research opportunities that still await researchers and designers in the person-environment transaction field.

* * *

One of the characters in Sartre's play *No Exit* declares that, "One always dies too soon or too late." I think that we all share the sentiment that Powell Lawton's death in January 2001 was premature. At the same time I feel privileged to have known him, and grateful to have spent time in the presence of someone who truly made the world a better place.

REFERENCES

Achenbaum, A. W. (1995). *Crossing frontiers: Gerontology emerges as a science.* New York: Cambridge University Press.

Altman, I., and Rogoff, B. (1987). *World views in psychology: Trait, interactional, organismic, and transactional perspectives.* In D. Stokols & I. Altman (Eds.), *Handbook of Environmental Psychology* (Vol. 1). New York: John Wiley.

Brody, E. M. (2000). Foreword. In R. L. Rubinstein, M. Moss, & M. H. Kleban (Eds.), *The many dimensions of aging.* New York: Springer Publishing Company.

Cohen, U., and Weisman, G. (1991*). Holding on to home: Designing environments for people with dementia.* Baltimore, MD: Johns Hopkins University Press.

Cohen, U., and Day, K. (1993). *Contemporary environments for people with dementia.* Baltimore, MD: Johns Hopkins University Press.

Golant, S. M. (1998). Changing an older person's shelter and care setting: A model to explain personal and environmental outcomes. In R. J. Scheidt & P.G. Windley (Eds.) *Environment and aging theory: A focus on housing.* Westport, CT: Greenwood Press.

Habraken, J. (1979). "Notes of a traveler." *Journal of Architectural Education*, 23, 4, 4-7.

Hacking, I. (1983). *Representing and intervening.* Cambridge, U.K.: Cambridge University Press.

Hamilton, D. (1994). Traditions, preferences, and posture in applied qualitative research. In N. K. Denzin and Y. S. Lincoln (Eds*.) Handbook of qualitative research.* Thousand Oaks, CA: Sage Publications.

Hedrick, T. E., Bickman, L., and Rog, D. J. (1993). *Applied research design: A practical guide.* Newbury Park, CA: Sage Publications.

Hillier, B. (1996). *Space is the machine.* New York: Cambridge University Press.

Hoglund, D., and Ledewitz, S. (1999). Designing to meet the needs of people with Alzheimer's disease. In B. Schwarz & R. Brent (Eds.), *Aging, autonomy and architecture: Advances in assisted living.* Baltimore, MD: The Johns Hopkins University Press.

Howell, S. C. (1980). *Designing for the aging: Patterns of use.* Cambridge, MA: The MIT Press.

Ittelson, W. H. (1973). *Environment and cognition.* New York: Seminar Press.

Kant, I. (1968). Analytic and synthetic judgment. In J. Margolis (Ed.), *An Introduction to Philosophical Inquiry.* New York: Knopf.

Kaplan, A. (1964). *The conduct of inquiry.* Scranton, PA: Chandler.

Kuhn, T. S. (1970). *The structure of scientific revolutions* (2nd ed.) Chicago: University of Chicago Press.

Lang, J. (1987). *Creating architectural theory: The role of the behavioral sciences in environmental design.* New York: Van Nostrand Reinhold.

Lawton, M.P. (1976). The relative impact of congregate and traditional housing on elderly tenants. *The Gerontologist,* 9, 15-19.

Lawton, M.P. (1980). *Environment and aging.* Belmont, CA: Brooks-Cole.

Lawton, M.P. (1982). Competence, environmental press, and adaptation. In M.P. Lawton, P.G. Windley, and T.O. Byerts (Eds.) *Aging and the environment.* New York: Springer.

Lawton, M.P. (1985). The elderly in context: Perspectives from environmental psychology and gerontology. *Environment and Behavior,* 17, 501-519.

Lawton, M.P. (1990). An environmental psychologist ages. In I. Altman & K. Christensen (Eds.) *Environment and behavior studies: Emergence of intellectual traditions.* New York: Plenum Press.

Lawton, M. P. (1990a). Knowledge resources and gaps in housing for the aged. In D. Tilson (Ed.) *Aging in place: Supporting the frail elderly in residential environments.* Glenview, IL: Scott, Foresman Professional Books on Aging.

Lawton, M.P. (1998). Environment and aging: Theory revisited. In R. J. Scheidt & P. G. Windley (Eds.) *Environment and aging theory: A focus on housing.* Westport, CT: Greenwood Press.

Lawton, M.P. (1999). Environmental taxonomy: Generalizations from research with older adults. In S. L. Friedman & T. D. Wachs (Eds.), *Measuring environment across the life span.* Washington, DC: American Psychological Association.

Lawton, M.P., and Nahemow, L. (1973). Ecology and the aging process. In C. Eisdorfer & M.P. Lawton (Eds.), *The psychology of adult development and aging* (pp. 619-674). Washington: American Psychological Association.

Lemke, S., and Moos, R.H. (2001). Residential alternatives for older Americans. *Journal of Architectural and Planning Research,* 18, 3, 194-207.

Nahemow, L. (2000). The Ecological Theory of Aging: Powell Lawton's Legacy. In R. L. Rubinstein, M. Moss, & M.H. Kleban (Eds.), *The many dimensions of aging.* New York, NY: Springer Publishing Company.

Parmelee, P.A., and Lawton, M.P. (1990). The design of special environments for the aged. In J.F. Birren and K.W. Schaie (Eds.) *Handbook of the psychology of aging* (3rd Edition). New York: Academic Press.

Patton, M. Q. (1990). *Qualitative evaluation and research methods.* (2nd Edition). Newbury Park, CA: Sage Publications.

Regnier, V., Hamilton, J., and Yatabe, S. (1995). *Assisted living for the frail: Innovations in design management, and financing.* New York: Columbia University Press.

Rouse, J. (1987*). Knowledge and Power: Toward a political philosophy of science.* Ithaca, NY: Cornell University Press.

Rubinstein, R. (1998). The Phenomenology of Housing for Older People. In R.J. Scheidt & P.G. Windley (Eds.) *Environment and aging theory: A focus on housing.* Westport, CT: Greenwood Press.

Rubinstein, R. L., Moss, M., and Kleban, M. (2000). Introduction. In R.L. Rubinstein, M. Moss, & M.H. Kleban (Eds.), *The many dimensions of aging.* New York: Springer Publishing Company.

Scheidt, R.J., and Windley, P.G. (1985). The ecology of aging. In J.E. Birren and K. W. Shaie (Eds.), *Handbook of the psychology of aging* (2nd Edition). New York: Van Nostrand Reinhold.

Scheidt, R.J., and Windley, P.G. (1998). Preface. In R. J. Scheidt & P.G. Windley (Eds.), *Environment and aging theory: A focus on housing.* Westport, CT: Greenwood Press.

Schwarz, B., and Brent, R. (Eds.). (1999). *Aging autonomy and architecture: Advances in assisted living.* Baltimore, MD: The Johns Hopkins University Press.

Turnbull, D. (2000). *Masons, tricksters and cartographers.* The Netherlands: Harwood Academic Publishers.

Wahl, H.W. (2001). Environmental influence on aging and behavior. In J.E. Birren and K.W. Schaie (Eds.) *Handbook of the psychology of aging* (5th edition). New York: Academic Press.

Zeisel, J., Epp, G., and Demos, S. (1978). *Low-rise housing for older people: Behavioral criteria for design.* Washington: Office of Policy Development and Research, U.S. Department of Housing and Urban Development.

Zeisel, J., Welch, P., Epp, G., and Demos, S. (1982). *Mid-rise elevator housing for older people.* Cambridge, MA: Building Diagnostics.

Vision and Values:
M. Powell Lawton
and the Philosophical Foundations
of Environment-Aging Studies

Gerald D. Weisman
Keith Diaz Moore

SUMMARY. As the formative figure in the emergence and development of Environment-Aging Studies, M. Powell Lawton influenced virtually every facet of this realm of research. Among his many
contributions, Lawton helped shape the philosophical foundations which
underlie the field and give direction to goals, theories, methods, and
strategies of research. These philosophical foundations of Environment-Behavior Studies are analyzed from five complementary perspectives–axiological, ontological, epistemological, methodological, and
praxeological–with particular attention paid to Lawton's position on
each. Though unwavering in his position with regard to values, Lawton
explored a variety of philosophical positions and continued to work to-

Gerald D. Weisman is affiliated with the University of Wisconsin-Milwaukee.
Keith Diaz Moore is affiliated with the Washington State University.
The authors were assisted in our task by former University of Wisconsin-Milwau-
kee colleague Habib Chaudhury, with whom we were honored to author a chapter
(Weisman, Chaudhury, & Diaz Moore, 2000) in *The Many Dimensions of Aging*
(Rubenstein, Moss, & Kleban, 2000), a festshrift prepared for Powell Lawton's 75th
birthday.

[Haworth co-indexing entry note]: "Vision and Values: M. Powell Lawton and the Philosophical Foundations of Environment-Aging Studies." Weisman, Gerald D., and Moore, Keith Diaz. Co-published simultaneously in *Journal of Housing for the Elderly* (The Haworth Press, Inc.) Vol. 17, No. 1/2, 2003, pp. 23-37;
and: *Physical Environments and Aging: Critical Contributions of M. Powell Lawton to Theory and Practice*
(ed: Rick J. Scheidt, and Paul G. Windley) The Haworth Press, Inc., 2003, pp. 23-37. Single or multiple copies
of this article are available for a fee from The Haworth Document Delivery Service [1-800-HAWORTH, 9:00
a.m. - 5:00 p.m. (EST). E-mail address: getinfo@haworthpressinc.com].

ward a meaningful synthesis of what are often seen as conflicting world-views. *[Article copies available for a fee from The Haworth Document Delivery Service: 1-800-HAWORTH. E-mail address: <getinfo@haworthpressinc.com> Website: <http://www.HaworthPress.com> © 2003 by The Haworth Press, Inc. All rights reserved.]*

KEYWORDS. Environment-behavior, paradigms, "good life" model, competence-press model

It is widely recognized that M. Powell Lawton played *the* formative role in the emergence and development of Environment-Aging Studies. As will be detailed by the other authors in this collection, Lawton's contributions were broad ranging, encompassing theory, method, and substantive research. Equally important, though perhaps less widely recognized, Lawton also made fundamental contributions to the philosophical foundations of Environment-Aging Studies. Thus, the task we have set for ourselves is the explication of a number of the key philosophical issues–sometimes more and sometimes less explicit in Lawton's writings–which have given shape not only to his own body of work but to Environment-Aging Studies more broadly. This is clearly a daunting assignment, one which only Lawton himself would have been truly equipped to take on. Fortunately Lawton, always extraordinarily generous in sharing his ideas and insights, has provided us with considerable guidance, most notably his chapter in the Scheidt and Windley volume (Scheidt & Windley, 1998) and an even more recent research proposal directed toward the development of a "lexicon" for the design of environments for dementia care.

We will examine the theoretical foundations of Environment-Aging Studies from five complementary perspectives that circumscribe the philosophical foundation of any paradigm: axiological; ontological; epistemological; methodological and praxeological (Moore, 1997). Collectively, these five perspectives capture the essential features of what Altman and Rogoff (1987) characterize as the "world views" underlying psychological research.

> These world views . . . are associated with different definitions of psychology and its units of study, different assumptions about the nature of person-environment relationships, varying conceptions about the philosophy and goals of science, and potentially different theories, methods, and strategies of research. (Altman & Rogoff, 1987, p. 7)

We conclude with brief consideration and conjecture regarding the philosophical directions–and the efforts to synthesize alternative world view–to be found in some of Lawton's final work. Such attempts at synthesis, and the challenges they present to Environment-Aging Studies, constitute yet another dimension of Powell Lawton's legacy.

AXIOLOGY

Axiology focuses on the study of the nature and types of values as well as appropriate criteria for values and value judgments. As we have previously asserted (Weisman, Chaudhury & Diaz Moore, 2000), Lawton, from the earliest days of his career, assumed a clear and principled position with respect to the place of values in Environment-Aging Studies. At a time when most social scientists believed–or perhaps hoped–that their research was value-free, and that the introduction of value positions tainted research validity, Lawton assumed a very different stance. More than two decades ago, he asserted that "the right to a decent environment is an inalienable right and requires no empirical justification" (Lawton, 1980, p. 160). His earliest theoretical formulation–the environmental docility hypothesis (Lawton & Simon, 1968)–focused on those individuals of lesser competence and the subsequent Ecological Model of Aging (Lawton, 1982) gave imagable visual expression to the differentially greater impact of environmental change upon the less competent (Figure 1).

As demonstrated by Nahemow (2000), these theoretical advances have proved to be a fruitful basis for both empirical inquiry and hypotheses generation; they illustrate the ways in which Lawton's creative mind was directed by his intrinsic value position. His work thus integrates both empirical and ethical bases of knowledge, demonstrating the ways in which each can, does, and must inform the other. More generally, the multifaceted nature of Lawton's work is a clear expression of the values underlying his belief that "theory, empirical research, service delivery, and policy develop in mutually reinforcing fashion" (Lawton, 1980, p. 164). In this phrase, Lawton reveals his true ambition for research that informs better practice–research focused on informing improvements in people's lives. It is this integration of ethics and empiricism that gives Lawton's diverse oeuvre its comforting coherence.

ONTOLOGY

Ontological concerns–analysis of the nature and relations of being and the question of what is *real*–loom large in Lawton's thinking and writing as well as in Environment-Aging Studies more generally. In considering the nature of the relationship between person and environment, Lawton notes what he char-

FIGURE 1. Lawton and Nahemow's Competence-Press Model

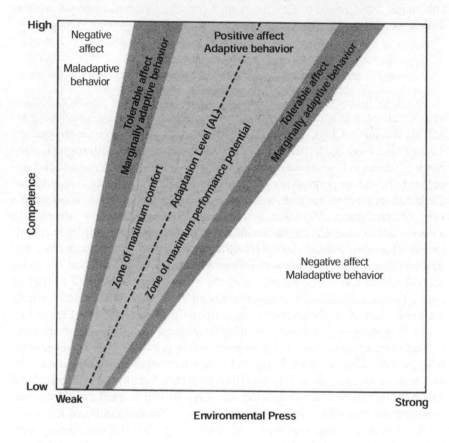

acterizes as a continuing "tension between holistic and separatist views of this interface" (Lawton, 1998, p. 1); this tension is clear in his own work and looms large as an issue in the field as a whole. Early on, Lawton (1980) laid out what may be characterized as a *separatist* position. While acknowledging the "intricate . . . continuously shifting and mutually causal" interchanges between person and environment, he concluded that "when one must operationalize, measure, and treat variables statistically, the problems become hopeless unless distinctions are made" (1980: 11). This separatist position was clearly reflected in Lawton's adaptation of Lewin's original ecological equation, B = f(P, E), with the addition of a P × E *interactional* term.

A decade later however, in their chapter of the *Handbook of the Psychology of Aging*, Parmalee and Lawton (1990) take what appears–at least at first glance–to be a very different perspective; they explicitly advocate a *holistic* or *transactional* approach as offering "the best opportunity to move the field (of Environment-Aging Studies) beyond its currently languishing state" (Parmalee & Lawton, p. 483). Finally, late in the 1990s, in his chapter in the Scheidt and Windley (1998) volume, it would seem that Lawton again returned to the initial separatist perspective of his early work.

> . . . although person and environment form a unified system where what is inside is philosophically inseparable from what is outside, for heuristic purposes, it is necessary to speak of, and attempt to measure them separately. (Lawton, 1998, p. 1)

Given this apparent oscillation, one might reasonably ask what constituted Lawton's "true" position on the relation between person and environment? Why was it seemingly difficult for him to hold to a single perspective over this period of roughly two decades?

While any response to these questions clearly involves more than a little conjecture, we believe that the beginnings of an answer are to be found in Lawton's "Good Life" (later "Quality of Life") model (Lawton, 1983). In this model, Lawton seemingly did not feel the need to *choose sides*, to assume either a separatist *or* a holistic perspective. The four overlapping circles of this well known diagram (Figure 2) represent both separate, directly measurable factors–specifically *objective environment* and *behavioral competence*–and two more holistic and integrative constructs–*psychological well being* and *perceived quality of life*. Most significantly, the center of the diagram–the point of overlap and integration of these four realms–is *the self*, the most holistic and integrative of psychological constructs. With the Quality of Life model, Lawton clearly had the courage to go where others chose not to tread, advocating a merging of what are traditionally viewed to be distinct if not conflicting ontological positions.

In one of his final research proposals, *An Environmental Design Lexicon for Dementia Care* (hereafter referred to as the Design Lexicon proposal), Lawton may have hinted at a strategy for synthesis of the *holistic-separatist* divide. Searching "for an alternative to the relatively rigid positivist approach," Lawton, in his proposal narrative, advocates building upon *The Pattern Language* of Christopher Alexander and colleagues (1977) "which sought scientific knowledge in systems and models, rather than cause and effect sequences" (Lawton, 1999, p. 5). Such an approach reflects key aspects of what Altman and Rogoff (1987) have characterized as an *organismic* or *systemic* world view, one which affords the capability of analyzing person × environment systems holistically *or* separately.

FIGURE 2. Lawton's Four Sectors of Quality of Life

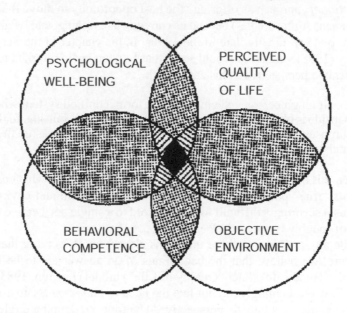

EPISTEMOLOGY

In posing the question, "What is the nature of knowledge?," epistemology is to a great extent shaped by one's ontological position. Within the separatist view of person-environment relationships, for example, the world is viewed as objective, and external to the person; the person in turn is viewed as a mechanism that responds to given stimuli presented by that eternal world. The nature of knowledge sought is thus defined in terms of generalizable cause-and-effect laws summarizing the relationships between objectively defined stimuli (independent variables) and observable responses (dependent variables). Such an effort requires identification of all salient variables and the ability to control those not under study. The person-environment system is viewed as being reducible; that is, the nature of relationships between any particular aspects of the system are not changed by controlling for or eliminating other parts of the overall system. Such ability to control and to reduce the person-environment system is essential for the generation of the cause-and-effect statements sought.

Conversely, the holistic view of person-environment relationships suggests that the person-environment system is completely integral and inseparable.

Knowledge sought within this viewpoint generally is comprised of subjective accounts of personal experience. Phenomenological inquiry, such as Rubinstein's (1989) inquiry into the meaning of home for the elderly, is reflective of such a holistic perspective. Knowledge is seen as subjective and local, revolving around integrative constructs such as meaning, self and experience.

As suggested above, Lawton viewed the separatist-holistic dialectic as something of a false dichotomy, recognizing that there are also socially-shared understandings. By way of example, Lawton's (1980) environmental taxonomy suggests four levels of human aggregation (individual, group, suprapersonal and societal) as well as three levels of environmental definition or conceptualization (physical, consensual, phenomenal). Consensually-held understandings are by definition shared at the group, suprapersonal and societal levels of aggregation, and thereby constitute meaningful levels of analysis in their own right. Here again, Lawton breaks down philosophical barriers, as well as traditional disciplinary boundaries defined by level of analysis.

Returning to the Quality of Life (QOL) model, Lawton (1983) integrates what have traditionally been considered mutually exclusive positions. The model allows for discrete aspects of QOL to be defined and operationalized, thereby facilitating separatist inquiry, while still incorporating the holistic concept of self, an ineffable construct best pursued holistically. It is a testament to his theoretical rigor that the different types of knowledge implied in his model are explicitly reflected in his definition of quality of life: "Quality of life is the multi-dimensional evaluation, by both intrapersonal (subjective) and social-normative criteria, of the person-environment system" (parentheses added) (Lawton, 1991, p. 6).

Of particular interest within the preceding quote is Lawton's hesitancy to articulate the traditional subjective-objective dialectic. Once one is willing to consider knowledge that is other than objective, the nature of knowledge becomes much more complex. As suggested above, the integral nature of person-environment relationships collapses epistemology and ontology, resulting in knowledge being socially-constructed. This presupposition is reflected in Lawton's use of the term *social-normative* and his definition of environment in physical, consensual, and phenomenal terms (Lawton, 1982).

Thus Lawton presents Environment-Aging Studies with the epistemological challenge of engaging in inquiry at multiple levels of analysis, tapping into subjective, consensual and objective ways of knowing. What form(s) might knowledge assume within such a perspective? Again Lawton's reference, in his Design Lexicon proposal, to *the pattern language* approach of Christopher Alexander et al. (1977) suggests an intriguing direction, albeit without providing definitive answers.

In brief, Alexander (1979) argues that people understand their world and the situations in which they find themselves in terms of *patterns*. One can think of a pattern in terms of three fundamental aspects: (1) a coherent system, constituted by the interrelationships between (2) components, which are (3) intentional (Merriam-Webster, 2001). In the context of Environment-Aging Studies, the system of interest is the person-environment system, characterized by Lawton (1980) as consisting of five components: the individual, group, suprapersonal, societal, and physical environments. Patterned thinking suggests that the interrelationships between these components are rooted in human intentionality. This is consistent with the concept of socially-constructed reality wherein people build their understanding of their world in relation to the goals they are seeking to advance, whether individually or collectively. This position within the theory of knowledge has been advocated by Berger and Luckmann (1966), Margolis (1987) and others. Fishman (1999) and particularly Polkinghorne (1992) have argued that patterned knowledge accords well with the tenets of neo-pragmatist philosophy, an approach we view as capable of accommodating the oscillations over time in Lawton's apparent ontological position.

METHODOLOGY

The preceding ontological and epistemological discussions seem to suggest that Lawton advocated a blending of positions previously viewed as mutually exclusive. Even his 1990 chapter, with its strong transactional emphasis (Parmalee and Lawton, 1990) advocated "a *mix* of qualitative and quantitative methods that allows person and environment to be measured both separately and transactionally" (emphasis added) (p. 5). Lawton's Design Lexicon proposal expresses a similarly inclusive attitude. "Although we by no means reject traditional positivism, we believe its advances will be fortified by our reports from the combination of qualitative and objective methods" (Lawton, 1999, p. 5).

At the same time it must be recognized and remembered that the assumptions guiding the conduct of inquiry clearly vary between those methods traditionally considered qualitative and quantitative. Lawton (1980) himself observed that "when one must operationalize, measure, and treat variables statistically, the problems become hopeless unless distinctions are made" (p. 11). These distinctions are made necessary in order to reduce the number of variables being examined in any given research study through the use of strategies which control for extrinsic variables, and often through statistical analysis and/or sampling procedures. Broadly speaking, most so-called quantitative methods adopt the "separatist" perspective discussed previously. The exemplar research design within the separatist perspective is the experiment with randomization and control groups. If certain procedures, methodological (e.g., random assignment) and analytical (e.g., matching data and statistical technique), are followed, the findings will be considered meaningful. Threats to validity (e.g., researcher bias) are carefully controlled, again through the use of agreed upon procedures. The more rigor there is to the procedures, or in other words the greater control and precision that is evident, the greater the power of statistical analysis that is possible. Greater statistical power in turn means the closer one gets to establishing cause-and-effect statements. Unfortunately for Environment-Aging research, such rudimentary aspects of the experiment such as control of environmental variables and random assignment of participants are often impossible in long term care and health care settings. It is for this reason that many environment-behavior studies involve correlational research which–while establishing the strength of relationships–remains, within the separatist perspective, a perceived poor second choice to the experiment.

Conversely, the transactional, or holistic perspective seeks an *ecologically-valid* setting, or in other words, a setting in which no control efforts are employed. In fact, a naturalistic context is essential to qualitative research, which views any control efforts as distorting the phenomena under study. While the separatist perspective assumes the phenomenon to be objective, with any researcher bias clearly to be eliminated, the holistic perspective accepts the inseparability of researcher and that being researched; the values of the researcher are expressed rather than suppressed. The holistic perspective seeks out themes and taxonomies that envelop a richness of data relationships, contrary to the separatist perspective that delimits the object of study to pre-defined variables.

Lawton's interest has always been to enhance the quality of living environments for the elderly by focusing on the relationships between people and the environment. This unabashed concern for the well-being of older persons creates a particular dilemma for the researcher engaged in experimental research which purports to forward objective, value-free findings. The need to reduce and control for a vast array of environmental variables within the experiment results in context stripping, and while increasing the paradigmatic rigor, Lawton seemed particularly troubled by its lack of relevance to decision-makers. While such research might produce broad generalizations, these might find little applicability in local situations–where action must take place. Quite simply, while Lawton felt quite willing to challenge traditional ontological and epistemological barriers, he would not betray his values.

As outlined in his Design Lexicon proposal (Lawton, 1999), understanding of the person-environment system requires multi-method research designs.

Subjective data should be collected, whether through interviews, diaries or an instrument like the Philadelphia Geriatric Center Affect Rating Scale (Lawton, Van Haitsma, & Klapper, 1996), the last of which Lawton referred to as a window on an intrapersonal phenomenon (affect). Objective data are not to be dismissed, and Lawton in fact suggests that such inquiry needs to be rooted in observation of human activity. Efforts should also be made to establish correlations with quantitative data garnered through various instruments as well as collecting "consensual" data of the kind represented by Moos and Lemke's (1996) measures of *social climate.*

Dealing with the resultant data types of data, varying in their source and type, gathered in relation to various levels of analysis, and addressing complex person-environment systems, clearly makes for a complex analysis. However, study of the *epistemology of practice* and neo-pragmatism (Polkinghorne, 1996) suggests that one particularly useful kind of knowledge to be derived from such analyses is in the form of patterns; as described previously, patterns have three aspects: intentions, components; and interrelationships. While the components of a system can be analyzed with descriptive data, interrelationships amongst components and the intentions that underlie those relationships must be interpreted. Intentions, once identified, may be assessed, with values immediately entering into the inquiry. Thus the all-too-frequent conflict over control between staff and residents in long-term care settings would likely be assessed differently by each group.

For these reasons, inquiry must be considered interpretive, with patterns emerging from interpretation of relationships between various components and the extent to which these patterns advance particular intentions. Patterns are never absolute; rather they continue to evolve as they strive to summarize one's best understanding of a given person-environment system at a given point in time. Time must be recognized as a powerful variable, as participants, the environment, intentions, and our very patterns of understanding continue to evolve.

PRAXEOLOGY

Praxeological considerations focus on assumptions about the relation between research and action. As noted by Moore (1997), one's view regarding the research-action interface is derived from one's axiology. Traditionally, behavioral science researchers have operated within what has been characterized as a *two-community* model (Min, 1987) where research and practice constitute two separate communities. The researcher's task is simply to develop knowledge and enhance the theoretical base; if research knowledge is implemented, it remains, within this model, the responsibility of *applied* researchers and practitioners. The *one-community* approach, by contrast, begins with the premise that the most applicable knowledge arises through the process of taking action to redress problematic, real-life situations; researchers are active participants in action-taking, either collaborating with practitioners or serving as the practitioners themselves. Echoing the *action research* perspective first postulated by Kurt Lewin, the one-community model utilizes theory, framed by a clear goal orientation, as the basis for action-taking and evaluation.

Given his underlying values, Lawton unquestioningly viewed Environment-Aging Studies research as working in the service of enhanced environmental quality for the elderly. While most of his work would seem to fall under the two community rubric, other projects–most notably his work on the Weiss Institute at the Philadelphia Geriatric Center–provide admirable examples of a one community approach.

The first skilled care environment specifically designed to address the needs of those with dementia, the Weiss Institute (see Figure 3), was planned with the explicit goal of "compensating wherever possible for the disorientation, memory loss, loss of social skills and sense of self typically demonstrated by organically brain damaged older persons" (Liebowitz, Lawton & Waldman, 1979, p. 59). The environment was viewed as a prosthetic, created to maximize competence in terms of individual orientation and socialization. This perspective led to a groundbreaking approach to nursing home design. With rooms arrayed around the perimeter of a large central space, Weiss Institute residents could survey all important activity areas from the thresholds of their rooms. It was intended that this immediacy of visual access would encourage participation in social activities occurring in the central space. Spatial orientation was facilitated by the central area serving as an orienting *landmark* and by color-coding of the thresholds to each resident room. Lawton was actively engaged in the several year planning effort (regular staff meetings, a national research conference) central to the implementation of the Weiss Institute.

Once completed and occupied, the Weiss Institute was the focus of an extended longitudinal evaluation study, with Lawton again the central figure (Lawton, Fulcomer & Kleban, 1984). The challenges presented by this evaluation study afforded Lawton yet another opportunity to comment on the tension between separatist and holistic perspectives. He was clearly frustrated at his inability to disentangle the many architectural and organizational features that collectively defined the Weiss Institute as experienced by its residents. "The independent variable itself was distressingly gross, in that the change in treatment locale subsumed *an immense variety of components whose effects are*

FIGURE 3. Floor Plan of the Weiss Institute

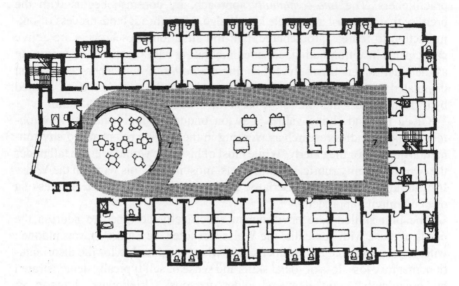

unquestionably related to one another in very complex ways" (Lawton et al., 1984, p. 755, emphasis added).

Precisely because the components of any person-environment system interact in complex, integrated ways, Lawton and his research team were unable to establish cause-and-effect relationships between specific features and resident behavior; nevertheless, the evaluation did find improvements with respect to overall project goals.

More generally, lessons from the Weiss Institute included new thinking in regard to the design of therapeutic environments for dementia care as well as implementation of the action-research model as a means for integrating research into the design process. The type of knowledge generated within such a one-community approach is likely structured in regard to a broad goal orientation and tends to focus on the complex interrelationships between the components of the person-environment system. It is interesting to note that a number of these shortcomings of the Weiss Institute evaluation were addressed in Lawton's subsequent conceptualization of Quality of Life. Here, the components of quality of life are viewed as mutually integrated yet separable in nature; subjective, consensual and objective approaches to knowledge–requiring utilization of a multiplicity of methods and the gathering of data from multiple perspectives–are all encompassed in Lawton's model. Coupled with a strong teleological base (found in its stress on the evaluation of quality), these features of the Quality of Life model may be seen as foreshadowing the pragmatic approach which begins to emerge in Lawton's Design Lexicon proposal. In his effort to better inform and reflect practical understanding, Lawton closes the circle from praxeology back to axiology.

CONCLUSIONS

Table 1 summarizes the several themes we have endeavored to sketch out with respect to the vision and values Powell Lawton brought to his own work, themes which have subsequently shaped the field of Environment-Aging Studies in significant ways. The rows of Table 1 describe the five complimentary philosophical questions of axiology, ontology, epistemology, methodology, and praxeology. The left and right hand columns represent the two oscillating world views–positivistic and phenomenological in character–reflected in Lawton's various ontological statements. The center column–something of a surmise on our part–represents which we believe to be an underlying philosophical perspective embedded in Lawton's Quality of Life model and in his endorsement of what we would characterize as a Pragmatic perspective in his Design Lexicon proposal. Review of the first row indicates a consistent and principled orientation to values. Ontology reflects the tension between separatist and holistic perspectives described above. Epistemology and Methodology follow from ontology; the former moving from a traditional positivist *cause-and-effect* approach to the search for consensually understood socially constructed patterns or relationships, to a transactional involvement in deeply rooted personal experience. Similarly methods move from the control of experiments or quasi-experiments, to multiple methods, to exclusively qualitative methods. Finally, praxeology finds itself oddly oscillating between first two-community, then one-community and back to two-community approaches.

In analyses such as those embedded in Table 1 we would do well to remember Altman and Rogoff's (1987) admonition regarding the validity and utility of world views.

> None of these world views provides the 'best' or 'correct' approach. They simply result in different forms of inquiry, understanding, and theory ... We ... advocate a complimentary use of alternative world views ... in order to avoid a doctrinaire, often ideological stance that there is an ultimate, true best, and correct way ... (p. 36)

TABLE 1. Comparison of the Separatist, Systemic and Holistic Perspectives

	Separatist	Systemic (Neo-Pragmatist)	Holistic
Axiology	• Decent Environment as Inalienable Right	• Decent Environment as Inalienable Right	• Decent Environment as Inalienable Right
Ontology	• World as External and Objective	• Social Construction	• Relativist Specific Realities
Epistemology	• Cause & Effect	• Patterns	• Experience
Methodology	• (Quasi) Experiment • Quantitative Methods	• Qualitative & Quantitative Methods	• Qualitative Methods
Praxeology	• Two-Community	• One-Community	• Two-Community

It is a tribute to M. Powell Lawton's own vision and values that he was able to avoid such doctrinaire, ideological perspectives in his own work and–through his own example–provide a rich, integrative, and deeply human philosophical foundation for Environment-Aging Studies.

REFERENCES

Alexander, C., Ishikawa, S. & Silverstein, M. (1977). *A pattern language.* New York: Oxford University Press.

Alexander, C. (1979). *The timeless way of building.* New York: Oxford University Press.

Altman, I. & Rogoff, B. (1987). World views in psychology: Trait, interactional, organismic, and transactional perspectives. In I. Altman & D. Stokols (Eds.), *Handbook of environmental psychology* (Volume 1, pp. 7-40). New York: Wiley.

Berger, P. & Luckmann, T. (1966). *The social construction of reality.* New York: Anchor Books.

Fishman, D. (1999). *The case for pragmatic psychology.* New York: University Press.

Lawton, M.P. (1980). *Environment and aging.* Belmont, CA: Brooks/Cole.

Lawton, M.P. (1982). Competence, environmental press, and the adaptation of older people. In M.P. Lawton, P. Windley & T. Byertss (Eds.), *Aging and the environment: Theoretical approaches.* New York: Springer.

Lawton, M.P. (1983). Environments and other determinants of well-being in older people. *Gerontologist, 23*, 349-357.

Lawton, M.P. (1991). A multidimensional view of quality of life in frail elders. In J. Birren, J. Lubben, J. Rowe & D. Deutchman (Eds.), *The concept and measurement of quality of life in the frail elderly* (pp. 4-27). San Diego: Academic Press

Lawton, M.P. (1998). Environment and aging: Theory revisited. In R. Scheidt & P. Windley (Eds.), *Environment and aging theory: A focus on housing.* Westport, CN: Greenwood Press.

Lawton, M.P. (1999). *An environmental design lexicon for dementia care.* Philadelphia, PA: Philadelphia Geriatric Center. Unpublished proposal.

Lawton, M.P., Fulcomer, M., & Kleban, M. (1984). Architecture for the mentally impaired. *Environment and Behavior, 16(6),* 730-757.

Lawton, M.P. & Simon, B. (1968). The ecology of social relationships in housing for the elderly. *The Gerontologist, 8*, 108-115.

Lawton, M.P., Van Haitsma, K. & Klapper, J. (1996). Observed affect in nursing home residents with Alzheimer's disease. *Journal of Gerontology*, 51B(1), P3-P14.

Liebowitz, B., Lawton, M.P. & Waldman, A. (1979). A prosthetically designed nursing home. *American Institute of Architects Journal*, 68, 59-61.

Margolis, H. (1987). *Patterns, thinking and cognition.* Chicago: University of Chicago Press.

Merriam-Webster Collegiate Dictionary (2001). *URL:http://www.m-w.com.*

Min, B.H. (1987). Relationship of strategic models and contexts to success of research utilization. Milwaukee, WI: Unpublished doctoral dissertation, Department of Architecture, University of Wisconsin-Milwaukee.

Moore, G.T. (1997). Toward environment-behaviour theories of the middle range: II. The analysis and evaluation of environment-behaviour theories. In T. Takahashi & Y. Nagasawa (Eds.) (1997). *Environment-behavior studies for the 21st century: Proceedings of the MERA 1997 International Conference.* Tokyo, Japan: University of Tokyo and Man-Environment Relations Association.

Moos, R. & Lemke, S. (1996). *Evaluating residential facilities: The multiphasic environmental assessment procedure.* Thousand Oaks, CA: Sage.

Nahemow, L. (2000). The ecological theory of aging: Powell Lawton's legacy. In R. Rubinstein, M. Moss & M. Kleban (Eds.), *The many dimensions of aging.* New York: Springer.

Parmalee, P. & Lawton, M.P. (1990). The design of special environments for the aged. In J. Birren & K.W. Schaie (Eds.), *Handbook of the psychology of aging.* San Diego, CA: Academic Press.

Polkinghorne, D. (1992). Postmodern epistemology of practice. In S. Kvale (Ed.), *Psychology and postmodernism.* Newbury Park, CA: Sage.

Rubinstein, R. (1989). The home environments of older people: A description of psychosocial processes linking person to place. *Journal of Gerontology*, 44, S45-S53.

Scheidt, R. & Windley, P. (1998). *Environment and aging theory: A focus on housing.* Westport, CN: Greenwood Press.

Weisman, G., Chaudhury, H. & Diaz Moore, K. (2000). Theory and practice of place: Toward an integrative model. In Rubenstein, Moos & Kleban (Eds.), *The many dimensions of aging.* New York: Springer.

Powell Lawton's Contributions to Purpose-Built Housing Design for the Elderly

Victor Regnier

SUMMARY. *Planning and Managing Housing for the Elderly* (1975) was an important book by Powell Lawton that established the foundation for many of the design guidelines and housing manuals that followed in the late seventies and early eighties. The data used to support advice and guidelines presented in the book were from a national evaluation of planned housing for the elderly conducted in the early 1970s. This work addressed a range of issues relating to location, design, and management. The approach to this book, which viewed planning and managing as a transactional partnership, influenced the way other researchers approached environmental design research. Today's environment-behavior research in gerontology owes much to Lawton's legacy of straightforward communication and practical insights. His ability to view research from a theoretical and applied perspective introduced an approach that has become an important teaching and communication strategy. *[Article copies available for a fee from The Haworth Document Delivery Service: 1-800-HAWORTH. E-mail address: <getinfo@haworthpressinc.com> Website: <http://www.HaworthPress.com> © 2003 by The Haworth Press, Inc. All rights reserved.]*

KEYWORDS. Purpose-built housing, housing policy, housing design, environmental support, adaptation

Victor Regnier is Professor of Architecture and Gerontology, University of Southern California, 10610 Lindbrook Drive, Los Angeles, CA 90024 (E-mail: regnier@usc.edu).

[Haworth co-indexing entry note]: "Powell Lawton's Contributions to Purpose-Built Housing Design for the Elderly." Regnier, Victor. Co-published simultaneously in *Journal of Housing for the Elderly* (The Haworth Press, Inc.) Vol. 17, No. 1/2, 2003, pp. 39-53; and: *Physical Environments and Aging: Critical Contributions of M. Powell Lawton to Theory and Practice* (ed: Rick J. Scheidt, and Paul G. Windley) The Haworth Press, Inc., 2003, pp. 39-53. Single or multiple copies of this article are available for a fee from The Haworth Document Delivery Service [1-800-HAWORTH, 9:00 a.m. - 5:00 p.m. (EST). E-mail address: getinfo@haworthpressinc.com].

INTRODUCTION

Lawton's contribution to the clinical gerontology literature and the theoretical literature on environment-behavior relations is well known. Perhaps less well-appreciated and less well known are his early insights regarding conceptual design, tenant management and site location characteristics of purpose-built housing for the elderly.

Between the mid-sixties and early seventies, great enthusiasm was focused on the social and behavioral aspects of architectural design. Organizations like EDRA (Environmental Design Research Association) were founded and the early Gerontological Society of America (GSA) project on Environment and Aging was initiated. Lawton was a founding member of the GSA project and was one of a handful of early EDRA participants. A major concern at that time was that environments for older people were being developed absent specific behaviorally based criteria. Furthermore, few post-occupancy evaluations were being conducted to pinpoint problematic features or identify successful features of purpose-built housing for the elderly.

Early publications in the aging literature, such as Francis Carp's analysis of Victoria Plaza (Carp, 1966), Pastalan and Carson's *Spatial Behavior of Older People*, and Irving Rosow's study of social patterns in apartment buildings (Rosow, 1967) as well as important publications like Newman's *Defensible Space* (1972) raised questions about the relationship between design decisions and social and behavioral outcomes. Beyond these studies little was directly applicable to design decision making. In fact, one of the first computer-based searches of the aging literature related to the planning and managing of housing (Regnier, 1975) revealed hundreds of publications related to this general area of study, but surprisingly few articles/books/reports focused on specific design considerations and recommendations. In the '70s architects seeking information about how design decisions affected the everyday life of older people, were relegated to either a painful search of the evaluative literature or reliance on codes that rarely focused on salient characteristics of the older person. The available literature included published buildings from architecture trade magazines or case study books (Musson & Heusinkveld, 1963; Rutherford & Holst, 1965). Neither of these sources reported on how well the building functioned after it was occupied.

The mid-seventies saw a flurry of books related to the general theme of design guidelines. Gelwicks and Newcomer's (1974) *Planning Housing Environments for the Elderly* resulted from the practical experiences and insights of two early housing pioneers. Another guidebook from the Michigan State Housing Development Authority (Green, Fedewa, Johnston, Jackson, &

Deardorff, 1975) detailed best practices which resulted from an examination of exemplary projects. However, Lawton's classic *Planning and Managing Housing for the Elderly* was the only publication that was comprehensive in nature and based on well-structured empiricism. It balanced technical information with data from research findings. Lawton also integrated his own practical experiences from the York House on the Philadelphia Geriatric Center's (PGC) campus. In 1980 Lawton published *Environment and Aging*, which summarized his perspective on the broader theoretical and applied considerations at that point. Chapters in this publication with design content focused on planned housing and institutions for the aged. In this publication he introduced many of his newest ideas on the design of housing for people with dementia. Again, actual experiences at the Weiss pavilion on the PGC campus informed his perspective about effective design interventions.

Lawton had a wonderful common-sensical, intuitive grasp of what was needed in housing. This was often modified and made more practical as a result of his emphasis on low-income housing. He was careful to identify priorities, make suggestions, and render judgments that led to the most powerful, cost-effective solutions. In the late 1960s, Lawton and his PGC colleagues received a grant that allowed them to evaluate one thousand Section 202 and public housing projects for the elderly. The outcomes of this research contributed much to the advice presented in this publication.

Lawton's insights were both practical and theoretical. They often resolved important questions but just as frequently raised other important questions and considerations. His thinking frequently examined architectural design within the context of neighborhood issues and management responsibilities. In short, he established the first set of empirically-based, thoughtful criteria oriented toward making the building more sensitive and responsive to older residents.

A number of important publications created in the wake of Lawton's work referenced his insights and built upon the need to more clearly identify answers to important questions. Research-based publications like Zeisel's *Low Rise Housing for Older People: Behavioral Criteria for Design* (Zeisel, Epp, & Demos, 1977) and *Mid-Rise Elevator Housing for Older People* (Zeisel, Welch, Epp, & Demos, 1983) explored many of the issues Lawton identified in a range of different housing forms.

Sandra Howell's analysis of common space and personal space use (Howell, 1980) and Koncelik's exploration of nursing home environments (Koncelik, 1976, 1982) introduced methodologies like behavior-mapping to more fully understand the use patterns associated with purpose built and institutional settings. In 1985, the American Institute of Architecture (AIA) created a guidebook (AIA, 1985) which attempted (although somewhat unsuccessfully) to

PHOTO 1. Book cover of *Planning and Managing Housing for the Elderly* (Lawton, 1975).

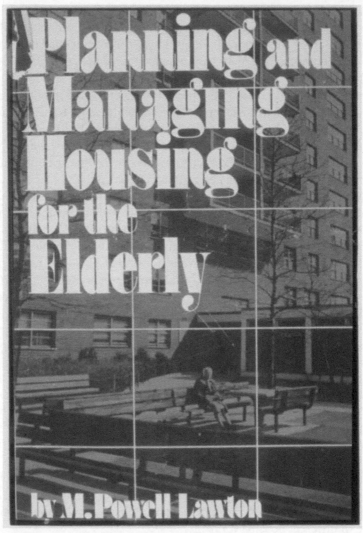

reconcile the range of guidelines which proliferated throughout the next decade. In editing the research based monograph *Housing for the Elderly: Design Directives and Policy Considerations*, our major goal was to collect the research insights of younger researchers who had all been influenced by Lawton's seminal work (Regnier & Pynoos, 1987).

PLANNING AND MANAGING HOUSING
FOR THE ELDERLY *REVISITED: REPRESENTATIVE ISSUES*

Lawton's (1975) *Planning and Managing Housing for the Elderly* is a 336-page book, subdivided into 14 chapters, the longest of which (102 pages) deals with "Designing the Building." Chapters are organized within three sections. The first section outlines issues related to the backgrounds of programs, principles, and people. The second part examines design, location, and planning considerations and the third part focuses on the role of management and services. The strength of the book resides in both its in-depth, highly detailed treatment of specific design considerations as well as its elucidation of broader issues affecting project conceptualization. The following ten issues are a representative sample of the considerations raised in the publication.

Supporting Personal Growth

Physical aspects of housing are relevant to the achievement of human goals in housing the elderly and society should provide environments that will challenge a person to produce one's best. Lawton recognized that a range of factors affected life satisfaction and well-being, but believed the environment was a significant influence. He identified two factors that affected satisfaction, particularly with older people. The first was the stress that the environment imposed on the individual. Lawton saw this stress having stronger impacts on older persons because of their diminished physical and cognitive capacities. Extreme cold or heat is difficult for everyone but particularly hard on older people because physiologically they cannot overcome this stress as easily as younger persons. He believed that "the older person in a large number of ways is more at the mercy of the environment than is a younger person" (Lawton, 1975, p. 56). In this way the environment could have a greater influence on the behavior of older people.

Lawton recognized the need for personal growth in older people and believed that often the environment didn't support this basic need. The desire to provoke curiosity, encourage exploration, and provide novelty are only a few of the ways the environment can be challenging and stimulating. In many cases, he believed that the need to explore was as strong as the need for security and designers should never allow the environment to patronize the older person or to limit the ability for self-initiated growth. The lack of opportunities for exercise is one of the most important opportunities often overlooked in contemporary environments. Residents need to feel challenged as much as they need to feel supported.

Prosthetic Environments and Adaptive Behavior

Another major goal is to provide prosthetic environments that will help maintain adaptive behavior in the less competent elderly. Lawton made a distinction between therapy and prothesis. He saw therapy as a treatment, which had the potential of changing the individual to overcome a functional deficit. Therapy would occur for a short time and when the individual was "cured," the therapy would cease. For example, penicillin can be used as a therapeutic response to an infection. However, for older people many of the conditions of aging don't lend themselves to therapeutic intervention because the conditions are chronic. For example, eyeglasses are prosthetic devices that allow the older person to see better. The same can be said for a leg brace that allows a person to walk or insulin that allows the diabetic to lead a full life. The total environment or a part of the environment can be designed to serve as a prosthesis. An elevator does this for a wheelchair resident in a multi-story building. Whereas another older person who wants to get exercise can use the stairs. Prostheses are best when they can be used individually but still provide choices for others. Older people are more likely to suffer from chronic conditions which increases the utility of prosthetic interventions.

Environmental Stimulation (versus Environmental Support)

One planning goal should be to provide residents with the widest range of environmental options to enrich and sustain life. Lawton's "environmental docility hypothesis" (Lawton and Nahemow, 1973) emphasizes the match between the person and the environment and its positive impact on a satisfying life. Most people (old and young) choose to "strike a balance between choosing an environment that is interesting (challenging, life-enriching) and one that is easy for him to live in (supportive, life-sustaining)" (Lawton, 1975, p. 61). There is great variability between older individuals; therefore the process of matching the person to the setting is one that must accommodate a range of different circumstances. In fact, as people age their need for more and different supports may occur. Therefore, the environment should be as adaptable as possible. Lawton believed the environment should always be slightly more challenging (or stimulating) than it is supporting. To add to the richness of this concept, Lawton used many metaphors. One of the most interesting which recognizes the dynamic nature of this match was the idea of taking a shower. We often start with one level of warmth but increase the water temperature as we become acclimated and desire more stimulation. Taking a shower is a dynamic balance of the environment (water temperature) and the individual's response.

The Management/Design Partnership

Management and design are transactional partners that depend on one another for maximum effect. Lawton was one of the first to perceive a transactional relationship between design and management. Both the style of management and the impact of services directed by management played a role in his thinking. This perspective called attention to management as a co-contributor of success. It is not enough to create a skillful design if it is poorly directed. The management of the environment had a profound impact on how well-satisfied residents were with their environments. He went on in the book to articulate criteria for selecting a good manager and to identify prevalent attitudes one might expect to encounter in potential candidates. Lawton knew the art of management was as important as an artful approach to design. He also encouraged us to seek individuals with appropriate attitudes. He felt that individuals could be trained to carry out technical jobs but if a new hire didn't have an affective bond with older residents, they would never be highly effective managers.

Optimizing Design Solutions

He rejected the stereotype of the designer as ego driven. Lawton believed that many past design mistakes were often misguided, innocent errors of judgment that failed to account for unforeseen side effects. He ascribed many bad practice judgments to lack of knowledge rather than a devious alternative personal agenda. In fact, he believed important design decisions which often had to be made with incomplete information, were great candidates for testable hypotheses in future research. His goal was to enfranchise designers with more knowledge about the side effects of various design decisions and to establish a hierarchy between minor and major considerations. In the long run, if architects could be educated about the broader issues at stake the building design would be more resilient. Lawton also understood the nature of design trade-offs and knew that optimizing a design solution meant that it would most likely never be a perfect solution. In fact, Lawton held the sponsor accountable for contributing to major decisions regarding the building program and design. This is one reason why *Planning and Managing* was written for a broader audience. He believed that both architects and providers should be well informed about the environmental choices available to older residents.

The Importance of Neighborhood Contexts

Neighborhood quality and location criteria were also considered critical to success. The success of any project is also partly dependent on the quality and supportive nature of the surrounding neighborhood. Independent housing that is isolated from stores, services, and public transportation is likely to flounder or fail. Furthermore, neighborhood security and the "defensible" nature of the building design also greatly affect residents' satisfaction and their perceived sense of control. For Lawton, environment was indistinguishable from the broader context of city and place. The orientation of the building, its connection to the street, and its ability to support outdoor recreational spaces all contribute to its success. After all residents who moved to age-segregated housing were often trading a broader set of community contacts for a more intimate group of friends and acquaintances. If the neighborhood was unfriendly or unsupportive, it further narrowed the fullness of life one could experience in this new setting. The selection of an appropriate neighborhood continues to be one of the most important decisions a sponsor can make. In market rate housing, it often assures the success or guarantees the failure of a project.

Older Residents as Nominal (versus Substantive) Clients

Public housing design was complicated by the lack of feedback from residents. Lawton recognized the difference between the nominal and substantive client. Older public housing residents were nominal clients that rarely provided feedback to designers. In subsidized housing there is also no market feedback to inform sponsors about the successful or unsuccessful attributes of a building. The substantive client was often the housing authority or the sponsoring agency. Unless they were involved in producing multiple projects, they did not see the benefit of commissioning an elaborate evaluation of their current project. To be effective, Lawton believed the sponsoring organization needed to "be the advocate for the (older) consumer" (Lawton, 1975, p. 120) and be fully cognizant of design shortcomings after occupancy. This is one reason why Lawton was a believer in post-occupancy evaluations. These more formal examinations of the environment can inform owners of their shortcomings. Solutions to these problems can be explored in future capital expenditures or can be the basis for making adjustments to a new building.

Housing Projects and Support for the Wider Community

Buildings have a broader responsibility to support residents, especially as the residents become more frail. The concept of the "accommodating building" was discussed in-depth in later evaluation analyses (Lawton, Greenbaum, and Liebowitz, 1980). However, the ability of the building to provide supportive services to people in the community as well as residents in the building was the focus of a full chapter detailing the role of "On-Site Services." Learning from his own experiences with York House and the experiences of Victoria Plaza, he was an advocate for providing services in buildings so they could benefit the broadest range of people in the local surrounding neighborhood. In fact he felt "it is simply not morally acceptable to build an ingrown program" (Lawton, 1975, p. 296). His major concern in this chapter was how sharing could take place without creating cliques and rifts between insiders and outsiders. One of the major differences between Northern European housing and U.S. housing (Regnier, 1994, 2002) is the attitude toward serving people in the neighborhood. In northern Europe most housing projects are linked to senior community centers that provide meals, personal care, and nursing services to a broader population. The deep subsidies available in U.S. public housing often limited residents to paying no more than 30% of their gross income for housing. The outcome of this policy was that people in subsidized buildings received deep subsidies while those in the neighborhood lived in sub-standard housing while paying higher rates. When subsidized buildings shared their resources with neighborhood residents, the situation became more equitable.

Triangulating Methods to Determine Preferences

Lawton advocated for both examining behavior as well as asking residents about preferences. Although much of the data Lawton gathered in his early evaluation studies was in an interview or self-report format, he also encouraged researchers to watch what older people did in certain circumstances. He recognized that what people say and what they do are often different and that a complete picture can only be assembled if both observation and interview data are gathered and cross-examined. In *Planning and Managing*, Lawton warns the reader to be careful about consumer psychology approaches that treat the building decisions like a choice between breakfast cereals. He also warns about the "depth psychology" approach which claimed it "could discover what kind of cigarette you might buy by asking whether you loved your mother" (Lawton, 1975, p. 120). He felt that an "updated watch on what people actually do" is a much more reliable indicator of what they would prefer. Of course, residents only use what is available to them. They are unlikely to cultivate flowers and vegetables if there are no garden plots available. So observational data need to be linked to other measures to fully comprehend the range of needs and desires.

Need for Unified Housing Policy

He believed in a unified housing policy but recognized the inherent weaknesses in current codes. Much of the first part of the book is devoted to a description of the many federal programs that at the time supported housing construction and development. Most of these programs had been suspended by the Nixon administration by the time this book was published. He recognized the end was near for this 30-year policy of construction but was pessimistic about the housing assistance program under consideration that supported individual renters with financial assistance. Lawton continued to advocate for a unified, aggressive federal housing policy that established quality standards and targets for housing production. This call was futile and decades later most subsidized housing programs have been continued subsumed by individual states.

With regard to federal regulations and guidelines for design and construction, Lawton felt efforts like the minimum property standards (MPS) were misguided. First of all, these guidelines rarely considered the needs and desires of older people. Little, if any, behavioral data were used to justify standards. Furthermore, standards under MPS were normally targeted toward the lowest acceptable minimums rather than embracing an optimal approach to design. Quality and innovation were rarely recognized.

Practical Advice

Ninety percent of the advice Lawton provided in *Planning and Managing* is just as relevant today as it was over 25 years ago. In fact some of it bears repeating because it may not be as commonly followed today as it was then.

Starting with issues relating to security, safety and emergency, Lawton stressed basic issues such as non-skid surfaces, conveniently located grab bars and general handicapped accessibility. Suggestions like a porte cochere overhang at the entry door, a single entry point and the use of "L" and "U" shaped building configurations for "self-monitored" security are commonly followed today.

Low fences that help to demarcate territory and discourage short cuts work were desirable but taller "hostile looking" fences made the building appear unsafe and institutional. His advice in this regard often focused on how security could be provided without sacrificing the friendly look of the building from the street. After all, housing should be inviting to friends and relatives.

He also took on tough questions (e.g., should housing for the elderly utilize a high-rise or low-rise design?). Lawton's research showed a moderately strong preference for low-rise living. However, he also discovered that the majority of residents who moved into a high-rise ended up strongly liking this arrangement.

With regard to unit size and configuration, he talked about the desire expressed by many residents living in efficiency apartments for a separate sleeping area where intimate possessions like bed clothes and dressing-table objects

PHOTO 2. The kneeling and bending over that was necessary to use the under-the-counter refrigerator represented some of the most negative feedback Lawton received from residents of planned housing (Lawton, 1975, p. 150, Figure #17). Photo by Sam Nocella.

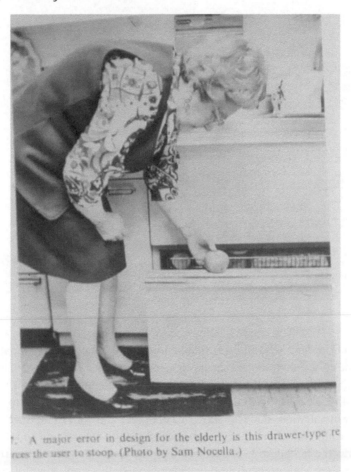

?. A major error in design for the elderly is this drawer-type re
rces the user to stoop. (Photo by Sam Nocella.)

can be kept out of the sight of visitors. Nearly a quarter of tenants living in studio units at PGC expressed that they would use part of a hypothetical income increase on a separate bedroom. Today, it is rare to find a new independent housing arrangement where more than 15% of the units are studios. Over the last 20 years we have seen a consistent increase in the size of independent housing units.

PHOTO 3. The porte cochere was lauded for its value in protecting residents as they moved from a car/bus to the front door of the building (Lawton, 1975, p. 178, Figure #37). Photo by Sam Nocella and building by Demchik and Supowitz, Philadelphia architects.

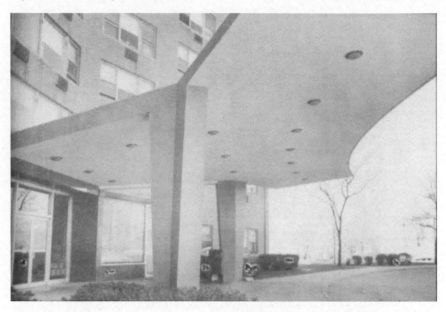

A section dealing with "self maintenance" underscores the impact that a poorly designed environment can have on independence. The topics of toileting, bathing, grooming, cooking, housekeeping, and sleeping are dealt with systematically. Features like outward swinging doors, toilets adjacent to walls for grab bar installations and pathways that are clear and well lighted are now frequently followed. One of the major findings in the assessment of kitchen designs was the unhappiness associated with the under-the-counter refrigerator. Residents who had to bend stoop or kneel to use this appliance found it very unsatisfactory. The warning about never having enough decentralized storage is a comment that could have come from a focus group discussion last week. Many of his predictions and judgments were very accurate, but a few missed the mark.

For example, there was a warning about the costly problem of providing a separate barber shop and beauty shop. He obviously missed the advent of gender-neutral hair cutting salons. Advice about the placement of ironing boards and the emphasis on hard surface tile in place of carpet, which at that time (carpet) was much more costly, seems a bit misplaced. His advice on emergency call buttons also seems a bit naive given the sophistication of today's communications systems. However, warnings about easy opening windows fell on deaf ears. Vinyl windows and tighter frames for energy and sound mitigation purposes have made it even more difficult to manipulate today's windows than the ones manufactured a quarter of a century ago. However, the emphasis on large windows and walking paths for exercise is excellent advice that has not been taken in enough new buildings today.

Interestingly, he could not find one building in the thousand he surveyed that had a "pet policy." Today nearly 70% of the assisted living buildings surveyed by ALFA (1999) allowed a "community pet" and given the influence of the Eden Alternative (Thomas, 1996) many nursing homes have come to see their benefits as well.

As an architect, I particularly appreciate his sensitivity to the beauty of the environment. He carefully explains the issue of how the environment affects an individual's self-assessment and advocates for color and pattern in furnishings, short corridors, and the use of balconies to add variety to the building's façade. His grasp of the importance of the building as a social context for friendship formation is stressed through comments about the strategic placement of social spaces and the need to accommodate a range of different social situations in the dining room. Nearly a dozen pages are devoted to programs, activities and social spaces that make the building a more animated and engaging place to live. He advocates for a variety of programs based on the past experiences and habits of tenants. Well before Howell's research (1980) on the design and placement of common space, Lawton advises that common spaces be conveniently placed in a central location near the elevator and the front door. He also warns us about the disadvantage of placing recreational activities on upper floors. Comments regarding the placement of outdoor benches and sitting areas reveal his observations about the attraction of activity and the need to provide security.

What was truly wonderful about Powell was his ability to bridge the gap between what he knew to be useful and what he felt was sensible given his extensive experience with the York apartments at PGC. A few of his personal and professional attitudes affected scores of colleagues.

EFFECTIVE LEADERSHIP AND PERSONAL CHARACTERISTICS

Lawton was always a person of action. He understood that we would never have all of the information to solve every immediate problem. However, we could use these problems as the basis for future research explorations. We served together on a design jury a few months before he became ill in July of 2001. He was, as always, interested in innovative practices that could make a difference in improving quality of life. He embraced the creative design process as a hypothesis establishing procedure that would ultimately help us to better understand the nature of any problem.

From the first encounter I had with Powell at a conference in 1971, I was always impressed with his passion for helping people. He helped others (and me) in countless professional ways and inspired me by his example to help others. In this regard he was an inspiration to all of us. I took a class he taught at the summer institute at USC in the early 1970s and I remember from that class his modesty and his enthusiasm in identifying with the passions of the students. Along with another student, I did a small study that replicated the work of Tom Byerts in recording how older people used outdoor seating in McArthur Park. Although it was not a part of the curriculum he envisioned, he adapted his classroom materials to our interests.

Powell was a wonderful facilitator who always seemed to look for ways in which he could help you. He went out of his way to help others by pushing opportunities in their direction. He was the strongest professional father figure I ever experienced. I felt like he treated me like a son. What surprised me most were conversations with Jerry Weisman and Graham Rowles about similar treatment. It is as though I have a collection of siblings who all benefited from his support, advice, and direction.

CONCLUSION

Because of my travel schedule I was on the East Coast in November, December and January of 2000 and had a chance to visit him in each of those last 3 months. He was aware of what could be done to extend his life. He had been around enough highly impaired people to know what was in store for him. His decision not to go ahead with treatment was about not being a burden to Faye, his wife, and to his children. A selfless, brave gesture that was so much like the M. Powell Lawton I knew.

REFERENCES

AIA. (1985). *Design for aging: An architect's guide.* Washington, DC: American Institute of Architecture (AIA) Press.

Assisted Living Federation of America (ALFA). (1999). *The assisted living industry, 1999: An overview.* Fairfax, VA: Price Water House Coopers and the National Investment Center.

Carp, F. M. (1966) *A future for the aged: The residents of Victoria Plaza.* Austin: University of Austin Press.

Gelwicks, L.E., & Newcomer, R.J. (1974). *Planning housing environments for the elderly.* Washington, DC: National Council on the Aging.

Green, I., Fedewa, B.E., Johnston, C.A., Jackson, W.M., & Deardorff, H.L. (1975). *Housing for the elderly: The development and design process.* New York: Van Nostrand-Reinhold.

Howell, S. (1980). *Designing for aging: Patterns of use.* Cambridge: MIT Press.

Koncelik, J. A. (1976) *Designing the open nursing home.* Pennsylvania: Dowden, Hutchinson and Ross.

Koncelik, J. A. (1982). *Aging and the product environment.* New York: Dowden, Hutchinson, and Ross.

Lawton, M.P. (1975). *Planning and managing housing for the elderly.* New York: John Wiley and Sons.

Lawton, M.P. (1980). *Environment and aging.* Monterey, CA: Brooks/Cole Publishing.

Lawton, M.P., Greenbaum, M. & Liebowitz, B. (1980) "The lifespan of housing environments for the aging." *The Gerontologist,* 20(1), 56-64.

Lawton, M. P., & Nahemow, L. (1973). "Ecology and the aging process," in C. Eisdorfer & M.P. Lawton (Eds.), *Psychology of adult development and aging* (pp. 619-674). Washington, DC: American Psychological Association.

Musson, N., & Heusinkveld, H. (1963) *Buildings for the elderly.* New York: Reinhold Publishing.

Newman, O. (1972). *Defensible space: Crime prevention through urban design.* New York: McMillan Press.

Pastalan, L. A., & Carson, D. (1970) *Spatial behavior of older people.* Ann Arbor, Michigan: University of Michigan Press.

Regnier, V., & Pynoos, J. (1987). *Housing the aged: Design directives and policy considerations.* New York: Elsevier Publishing.

Regnier, V. (1975). *Planning housing and services for the elderly: A bibliography.* Los Angeles, CA: Andrus Gerontology Center, University of Southern California.

Regnier, V. (1994). *Assisted living housing for the elderly: Design innovations from the United States and Europe.* New York: Wiley.

Regnier, V. (2002) *Design for assisted living: Guidelines for housing the mentally and physically frail.* New York: Wiley.

Rosow, I. (1967). *Social integration of aged.* New York: Free Press.

Rutherford, R.B., & Holst, A. (1965) *Architectural designs homes for the aged: The European Approach.* Peoria, IL: Howard Company.

Thomas, W. (1996). *Life worth living: How someone you love can still enjoy life in a nursing home?* Acton, MA: VanderWyk and Burnham.

Zeisel, J., Epp, G., & Demos, S. (1977). *Low-rise housing for older people: Behavioral criteria for design* (HUD Publication # 483). Washington, DC: USGPO.

Zeisel, J., Welch, P., Epp, G., & Demos, S. (1983) *Mid-rise elevator housing for older people.* Boston, MA: Building Diagnostics.

Many Meanings of Community:
Contributions of M. Powell Lawton

Rick J. Scheidt
Carolyn Norris-Baker

SUMMARY. Powell Lawton's theoretical and empirical work greatly increased understanding of communities as contexts for successful aging. This article illustrates the direct and indirect contributions of Lawton's work for multiple meanings of community at the physical, personal, suprapersonal, and social environmental levels. This includes the ETA (Ecological Theory of Aging) and its value as an empirical and practical tool for understanding environmental coping among old community residents; his seminal work on community planning; emotion as a determinant, moderator, and outcome of environmental adjustment, place identity, and place attachment in community settings; and his novel use of the dimension of time in community studies. We share some personal memories of the range and impact of Lawton's work and advice on our own community level research. *[Article copies available for a fee from The Haworth Document Delivery Service: 1-800-HAWORTH. E-mail address: <getinfo@haworthpressinc.com> Website: <http://www.HaworthPress.com> © 2003 by The Haworth Press, Inc. All rights reserved.]*

KEYWORDS. Communities, ecological theory of aging, community planning, emotion and place, time

Rick J. Scheidt and Carolyn Norris-Baker are affiliated with Kansas State University.

[Haworth co-indexing entry note]: "Many Meanings of Community: Contributions of M. Powell Lawton." Scheidt, Rick J., and Norris-Baker, Carolyn. Co-published simultaneously in *Journal of Housing for the Elderly* (The Haworth Press, Inc.) Vol. 17, No. 1/2, 2003, pp. 55-66; and: *Physical Environments and Aging: Critical Contributions of M. Powell Lawton to Theory and Practice* (ed: Rick J. Scheidt, and Paul G. Windley) The Haworth Press, Inc., 2003, pp. 55-66. Single or multiple copies of this article are available for a fee from The Haworth Document Delivery Service [1-800-HAWORTH, 9:00 a.m. - 5:00 p.m. (EST). E-mail address: getinfo@haworthpressinc.com].

In an autobiography written shortly before his death, Powell Lawton described the "threads that laced together the disordered sections" of his life (Lawton, 2000, p. 186). He discussed the pleasures he gained from experiencing the large-scale built environment, whether "the sense of newness in each configuration of buildings, pedestrians, stores, and greenery" in his first exploration of Pittsburgh's Golden Triangle, great cities like St. Petersburg or Sydney, "a new section of northeast Philadelphia or a small town like Moodus, Connecticut" (Lawton, 2000, p. 186). He wrote:

> Another facet of large-scale environmental experiencing comes when caring for the several acres of land on which we live. It is heavily wooded, hilly, and threatens to return to a scrub-growth and honeysuckle jungle if not persistently tamed. Cutting wood and brush and walking through the changing forest is my type of outdoor work, not small-plot gardening or lawn manicure. (Lawton, 2000, p. 186)

This statement serves as nice metaphor that distinguishes Powell's work orientation from that of most others. While he made major contributions to the specific components of the ecological equation, Powell Lawton was not a "small-plot gardener." He was a "writ-large" overseer in environment-aging studies. His view of the whole and his personal grace made him an invaluable colleague and mentor and a generous resource and friend to so many here today.

Community carried many meanings in his work. Lawton's thinking and research–to use his own taxonomy–examined community alternatively as part of the physical, personal, suprapersonal, and social environments (Lawton, 1999). As early as 1976, his conceptualization of community planning encompassed not only traditional issues such as housing, institutions, resource locations, transportation, geography and mobility, but physical and social planning and policy decisions, such as community services and programmatic aspects of senior housing, that directly affect the lifestyles and well-being of older citizens (Lawton, Newcomer, & Byerts, 1976). His objective was always to identify community alternatives and dimensions that enabled older residents to maintain their lifestyles as community dwellers and avoid institutionalization (Lawton, 1981b). The task of community planners, then, was to provide community settings and services congruent with the needs and expectations of older residents.

The practical focus of much of this work is represented by and partially derived from the Ecological Theory of Aging (Lawton & Nahemow, 1973), which he developed with Lucille Nahemow, who, sadly, also died quite recently. At the heart of the ETA was an early practical concern with configuring the environment–in various domains and levels–to support residential living within a noninstitutional community context (Nahemow, 2000) and, later, to bring the physical and social features of community to adult care settings (Newcomer, 2000).

The ETA model is a conceptual cornerstone of differential gerontology in environment-aging studies. It actively models individual differences in adaptation among a wide range of older community residents–represented, for example, in the "environmental docility hypothesis" (where changes in objective press levels disproportionately affect those with lower competence) and the "environmental proactivity hypothesis" (where a larger number of environmental resources are available to those who are more highly competent). It treats environment as a complex and interrelated set of physical and social attributes ranging from the micro-environmental to suprapersonal levels, and includes both objective and subjective dimensions of press. A research study by La Gory, Ward, and Sherman (1985) demonstrates the importance of this complex, multi-dimensional conceptualization of environmental press. When they studied a large representative group of community-dwelling older adults, they concluded that subjective, rather than objective, environmental press accounted for most of the variance in neighborhood satisfaction. Furthermore, "Older persons sharing the same neighborhoods do not necessarily occupy the same environmental worlds" (p. 405).

Studies of the environmental contexts in which frail community-dwelling elders reside and the processes marking both proactive and reactive responses to personal and environmental changes illustrate the importance of ETA as a foundation for community assessment and planning. They also illustrates the diverse individual competencies and preferences within any one community. In an article entitled "The elderly in context: Perspectives from environmental psychology and gerontology," Lawton points out that "getting to know one's environment is an active process of cognitive restructuring," and that this "residential knowing" is simultaneously a source of security and autonomy (Lawton, 1985, p. 508). The more an older person knows about the environment, the less its perceived press; and more autonomy is possible for a given level of competence. The longer an older person has resided in a dwelling and community, and the more stable the environment, the greater the experience and knowledge: ". . . one gets to know how to find neighborhood resources, how to use transportation, and who one's friends and neighbors are" (p. 508). The degree of challenge perceived in moving to a different residence and having to "learn" a new neighborhood or even community is often given as a reason not to move, even from an undesirable neighborhood (Lawton, 1986).

In a related example, Lawton describes community-dwelling frail elders who create "control centers" within their homes as a response to decreasing behavioral competence (Lawton, 1985). The importance of maintaining involvement with community is demonstrated by the location of these centers (usually a chair) in a place that provides a view of the house entrance and sidewalk, as well as easy access to telephone and television. Although these elders have relatively low levels of behavioral competence, they have gained increased security and control by restricting their range of physical and behavioral space. By continuing to be community residents, they are able to maintain valuable psychological autonomy. They are able to maintain "the idea that they still occupy their long-standing home, that they still live in their old neighborhood, and they are autonomous people living in the community, not in a dependent situation" (p. 516). Lawton's observations highlight his continuing focus on the importance of community characteristics and services for the well-being of older adults, balanced by an appreciation of the importance of wide individual variations in competence and perceptions of the environment.

COMMUNITY PLANNING

Community planning was a central feature of Lawton's thinking and research for many decades. Lawton was part of an early generation of influential researchers—including Fran Carp, Sandy Howell, Eva Kahana, Lee Pastalan, Irv Rosow, and Sylvia Sherwood—who initiated research to examine how elderly populations were affected by public policies governing urban renewal (Newcomer, 2000). He engaged in both observations and large-scale surveys of ecological characteristics of neighborhoods (Lawton, 2000). Lawton viewed this part of his career as "spirituality in action"–motivated by the concern of social policy makers with the directions that national housing programs should move. This included their thirst for knowledge regarding age segregation, ethnic mixing, housing-based services, fear of crime, as well as qualities of the physical environment (Lawton, 2000, pp. 191-192).

Newcomer (2000) charts the evolution of these efforts and their enormous influence on his own work and the work of others, such as Victor Regnier. Lawton's early work aided the development of

> A research-based understanding of physical design and how this could influence the quality of life of low-income elderly housing project residents, as well as the effects on elderly residents in low income minority neighborhoods. From this narrow beginning there eventually grew work that looked at transportation, neighborhood use, the changing age-mix of neighborhoods, and a vast understanding of the specialized housing needs of individuals with varying levels of functional and cognitive ability. (Newcomer, 2000, p. 241)

Lawton maintained a long-term concern with identifying the fundamental characteristics of community important to older adults. Investigations in the late 1970s led to the development of a scale of Perceived Community Function (PCF) which assesses attributes that contribute to residents' well-being and ways in which these attributes can satisfy residents' needs (Blake, Lawton, & Lau, 1978; Blake & Lawton, 1980, Lawton, 1986), thus indicating ways in which a particular community can plan for meeting its specific needs. In the research, older and younger adults described characteristics of an ideal community and evaluated their satisfaction with their own community based on many of those characteristics. The findings identified substantial agreement on the most important community attributes across age groups and for different size communities, ranging from large cities to small towns. The researchers were able to group the community attributes into three dimensions previously proposed by Insel and Moos (1974): (1) system maintenance (high quality medical care, schools, good jobs, and a wide variety of stores and businesses), followed in importance by (2) relationship to others (being near friends and relatives, having a voice in community affairs), and, finally, (3) personal development (recreation, entertainment, social organizations). Although older and younger adults ranked these attributes in similar orders, older adults assigned greater absolute levels of importance to items such as medical care and relationships to others. This pattern was attributed to the changing needs of the older adults and the community's ability to meet those needs (Lawton, 1986).

The book, *Community Planning for an Aging Society* (Lawton, Newcomer, & Byerts, 1976), integrated human service and planning issues and focused on ways that planning decisions affected the lifestyles of older people. A later volume, *Housing an Aging Society* (Newcomer, Lawton, & Byerts, 1986), treated housing as a service component, sensitized housing specialists to changing health and social service milieu, emphasized the influences of public policy and demography, and brought more attention to neighborhood and community contexts (Newcomer, p. 245). This work built partially upon Lawton's earlier (and now classic) considerations of community supports for the aged (Lawton, 1981a, 1981b), where both support and challenge dimensions of alternative residential choices were linked to characteristics of residents with varying levels of need.

Similarly, a chapter in Lawton's *Environment and Aging* (1986) was devoted to attributes of the macroenvironment, including neighborhood and community issues. Challenges listed for planners and service providers included:

1. locating people near desirable resources,
2. locating desirable services near existing concentrations of older adults,

3. mobilizing existing resources to provide more elderly-specific programs,
4. mobilizing informal neighborhood resources to support frail elders (neighborhood watch programs, friendly visitors, etc.), and
5. providing transportation to services or making services portable to serve elders who are unable to travel.

The legacy of these efforts can be seen in many venues, including environmental impact statements that include the evaluation of the appropriateness of projects and site locations in terms of potential residents and their neighborhood use needs. Other examples of lasting impact can be found in both research and public policy initiatives to identify communities already possessing or seeking to develop the attributes most important to particular groups of older adults, such as naturally occurring retirement communities (NORCs) and recreational/leisure communities.

Years later, Lawton noted with some regret that while this housing and community planning research benefited environmental design research and curricula development, a number of social issues in that research were neglected as "housing the poor" lost its political appeal (Lawton, 2000). "Social and service programs for the 700,000 older people living in these now-old (federal) housing projects are difficult to support, and this major need group has become a lost generation" (Lawton, 2000, p. 192). It remains for the next generations of researchers, community planners, and policy makers to redress this neglect.

Lawton also made a number of finer-grained contributions to our knowledge about senior housing. He examined housing transitions for both voluntary and involuntary moves. He used quasi-experimental comparisons among older community residents and those who moved to planned senior housing, using mortality and morbidity outcome rates with early results indicating relocation is helpful for some, stressful for others (Lawton, 1970). He argued for the balanced improvement of both institutional and community care systems, recognized that community care could not be a large-scale substitute for institutional care, and alerted us to the fact that a significant proportion of institutionalized elders could live elsewhere, with appropriate alternative housing (Lawton, 1978). More recently, he focused on caregiving for community elders, emphasizing new programs that provide psychological benefits for caregivers, calling for evaluation research to identify high risk caregiver groups, and advocated the integration of public and private payer systems around the central role of the family, under the umbrella of a single community agency (Lawton, 1996).

EMOTION AND PLACE

His later work also took him into the Environmental (E) and Person (P) components of the transactional ETA equation in greater depth. He expressed concern that individual needs and preferences, based on temperament and personality as well as functional abilities, would be lost among abstract generalizations such as security or autonomy related to housing (Lawton, 1998). He gave fresh thought to the taxonomic environment (Lawton, 1999) and, following career-long interests in clinical and personality issues, moved into the realm of emotion in aging–exploring "different action patterns of positive and negative feelings" (Lawton, 2000, p. 192). This work produced several measures designed "to tailor measures of familiar phenomena to the special situations of older people" (Lawton, 2000, p. 192). In looking back on his own research, he concluded that "there has been a strong tendency for positive emotional states to occur in older people who are more engaged with other people, leisure activities, and their environments" (p. 103). Thus a challenge for communities of all sizes is to provide older residents the appropriate opportunities for social and leisure pursuits to meet their needs, as well as environments and services that encourage proactive responses to changes in competence.

The outcomes of this work also complement his earlier premise that we know little about how well-being is related to "community as a 'place'," but that ". . . symbolic elements of attachment to a community . . . are worthy of study" (Lawton, 1986, p. 37). Parmalee and Rubinstein, both colleagues of Lawton, make personal identity central to place attachment for older adults, framing both local relocation and migration decisions (e.g., changing the E component) as decisions that directly pertain to self-identity (Rubinstein & Parmalee, 1992). Thus, concepts such as place meaning and place attachment can be encompassed within the ETA model. At the community level, strong emotional attachments may take varied forms, depending on individual differences in sense of place (Hummon, 1992). Community identity may provide some individuals with a sense of belonging and to derive some aspects of their own self-imagery as a type of person from community imagery (Hummon, 1986). Relocation, which can make major changes in environmental press, may involve reinterpretation of past place identities and changes in the roles in which an individual engages in community settings (Cuba, 1989). As a consequence, place attachment strengthened over long periods in a particular home and community may contribute to sustaining psychological autonomy as well.

TIME: THE FOURTH DIMENSION

We have long had a fascination with Powell's focus on time as a research dimension, on the evaluation and use of time in community settings. Time appears early in his work as the fourth component of the ETA (in addition to P, E, and Adaptation) and may be its most overlooked feature (Nahemow, 2000).

Lawton inserted time directly in his operational definition of the "behavioral day." In the spirit of Roger Barker's research on behavior settings (Barker & Wright, 1951), Lawton and Moss asked urban elders in four different community groups (community residents, public housing tenants; recipients of intensive in-home services; and an institutional waiting list group) to account for one full day using time budgets or "yesterday interviews." Days were recounted in 15 minute segments. These were coded for content, duration, social and environmental context, and the amount of liking for each activity. [The results are secondary to the central point, but care groups engaged in activities far less to their liking than the community group, which found itself engaging in more obligatory activities across a wider niche breadth (Moss & Lawton, 1982).]

This additional dimension of time is useful not only when applying the ETA to groups of individuals, but to the community dimensions of environmental press as well. Time provides not only cross-sectional measures of how activities or behaviors are allocated, but longitudinal documentation of changes in both patterns of time allocation and in both the P and E components of the model. Just as behavioral competence may increase or decrease for a given individual over time, a community's attributes are seldom constant, and aspects of environmental press may change irrespective of those in behavioral competence. Such changes at the community level are particularly important, because the impact extends to the environmental press experienced by many older adults. One example is the number and diversity of community settings and services available to an older individual. While these amenities and services may expand or contract over time, losses may have the greatest impact on press. Long-term patterns of decline over time are especially of concern in smaller communities and rural areas, where the loss of services (such as a health care setting, bank, etc.) or amenities are not easily replaced. Another aspect of the suprapersonal environment whose changes over time have been studied extensively is aggregate age structure of neighborhoods and communities. In addition to the studies of relocation and demographic patterns, the particular age structure of the community may influence the opportunities for social interaction, or even the availability of services and amenities, such as the case of naturally occurring retirement communities.

About ten years ago, Powell and Miriam Moss and Allen Glicksman used satisfaction with time as an indicator of perceived quality of life in The Good Life model. They compared the quality of the Last Year of Life (LYOL) of recently deceased elders to an ordinary year of life among a matched sample of older community residents–a very novel study. Declines in competence and well-being were reported for those in the LYOL group prior to their entrance into that last year (Lawton, Moss, & Glicksman, 1990).

The Valuation of Life (VOL) scale has roots in this research. This scale beautifully illustrates Powell's self-confessed search for novelty and the large picture in his measurement work (Lawton, 2000), giving us insight into how much older people value their lives–helping us understand "how people may cling to life or welcome its end" (Lawton, Moss, Hoffman, Grant, Ten-Have, & Kleban, 1999, p. 406). Valuation of Life is "the extent to which the person is attached to his or her present life, for reasons related to a sense not only of enjoyment and the absence of distress, but also hope, futurity, purpose, meaningfulness, persistence and self-efficacy," where "both environmental and personal factors, positive and negative features, and physical and mental health and pathology, all processed by the individual, jointly determine how much people value their lives" (Lawton, Moss, Hoffman, Grant, Ten-Have, & Kleban, 1999, p. 406).

ON RANGE AND NOVELTY

Like so many others, we are struck by the range and novelty of Lawton's work and by the fact that his footprints were among the first on so many new beaches. We would like to illustrate some of his community-oriented work with some personal observations.

Several years ago, Paul Windley and I (Scheidt) asked Lawton to serve as a consultant on a federally-funded project examining environmental predictors of the well-being of rural elders. He advised us to include hard measures of the physical environment in the study, and to dedicate a domain to satisfaction with community services. He consulted on measures of psychological status, several environmental domains, the training of interviewers, and offered a comparative data set from his PGC studies. We were very interested in how specific community attributes predicted to levels and types of well-being among our Kansas elders. Of course, we learned that Lawton had just collaborated in this area–developing the model of Perceived Community Functions (PCF) with Brian Blake in a rural Indiana county (Blake & Lawton, 1980.) From his vantage point in Philadelphia, Powell was conducting rural community research! We blended some indicators of the PCF approach within our measures of the psychological environment and it proved quite useful.

Powell also had a remarkable talent for synthesizing diverse ideas from his vast range of knowledge in unique ways. An example is his extrapolation of our (Scheidt & Norris-Baker) more recent work on "place therapy" and "behavior setting therapy" at the community level to planned and unplanned housing environments. We focused on ways in which communities, especially those threatened with loss of settings, might restructure their settings to sustain the services and activities needed by older residents and search for a different community identity, such as a recreational town or a bedroom community (Scheidt & Norris-Baker, 1999). Powell perceived the opportunities for applying the same concepts in housing environments as well as communities. He observed that:

> Their standing patterns of behavior may or may not facilitate the most adaptive or satisfying behaviors for the majority of occupants, or the standing pattern may suit the majority but be maladaptive or aversive for some individuals. As aging in place occurs, the rules that govern the standing patterns of behavior may need to be modified deliberately–for example, persuading the tenant group to accept people in wheelchairs in the lobby or dining room. (Lawton, 1998, p. 26)

Powell enjoyed developing unique methods that would reveal eco-behavior in new ways–including methods for sampling rare populations, the use of medical records as sampling frames and data sources, survey research on older minority adults, and longitudinal changes in subjects, methods, and environments (Lawton & Herzog, 1988; Lawton, 1987). He enjoyed immensely "working out the methodology for 'behavior maps' of institutional and housing environments and observational surveys of the ecological character of neighborhoods" (Lawton, 2000, p. 189).

CLOSING COMMENT

In the near future, environment-aging studies will continue to be influenced by the entire body of Lawton's work. The future of this field concerned him a great deal. He believed that we should place priority on the creative idea in environment-aging studies (Lawton, 2000), on new paradigms and methods. As Lawton himself indicated, creating environmental change at the community level is difficult (Lawton, 1998). While obviously respecting the power of environmental design, he believed strongly that we should also consider where, when, and how to change individual behavior–including teaching and taking lessons from older adults on how to do this. Powell Lawton's passing poses questions for the longer outlook: who will signal the value of these differences in the future, respect practice and research with equal fervor, move with ease among all components of the ecological equation, exhibit balanced comfort with theory and method, offer us a view far beyond the small garden plots, and grow new generations of researchers to tend our communities?

REFERENCES

Barker, R., & Wright, H. (1951). *One boy's day.* New York: Harper & Row.

Blake, B., & Lawton, M. P. (1980). Perceived community functions and the rural elderly. *Educational Gerontology,* 5 (4), 375-386.

Blake, B. F., Lawton, M. P., & Lau, S. (1978). *Community resources and need satisfaction: An age comparison.* Philadelphia: Philadelphia Geriatric Center.

Cuba, L. (1989). Retiring to vacationland: From visitor to resident. *Generations,* 13, 63-69.

Hummon, D. (1986). City mouse, country mouse: The persistence of community identity. *Qualitative Sociology,* 9, 3-25.

Hummon, D. (1992). Community attachment: Local sentiment and sense of place. In I. Altman & S. Low (Eds.), *Place attachment* (pp. 253-279). New York: Plenum.

Insel, P. & Moos, R. (1974). Psychological environments: Expanding the scope of human ecology. *American Psychologist,* 29, 179-189.

La Gory, M., Ward, R., & Sherman, S. (1985). The ecology of aging: Neighborhood satisfaction in an older population. *Sociological Quarterly,* 26, 405-418.

Lawton, M. P. (2000). Chance and choice make a good life. In J. E. Birren & J. F. Schroots (Eds.), *A history of geropsychology in autobiography* (pp. 185-196). Washington, D. C.: American Psychological Association.

Lawton, M. P. (1999). Environmental taxonomy: Generalizations from research with older adults. In S. Friedman & T. Wachs (Eds.), *Measuring environment across the life span: Emerging methods and concepts* (pp. 91-124). Washington, D. C. : American Psychological Association.

Lawton, M. P. (1998). Environment and aging: Theory revisited. In R. J. Scheidt & P. G. Windley (Eds.), *Environment and aging theory* (pp. 1-32). Westport, CT: Greenwood Press.

Lawton, M. P. (1996). Aging family in a multigenerational perspective. In G. H. Singer, L. Powers, & A. Olson (Eds.), *Redefining family support: Innovations in public-private partnerships* (pp. 135-149). Baltimore, MD: Brookes Publishing Company.

Lawton, M. P. (1987). Methods in environmental research with older people. In R. Bechtel, R. Marans, & W. Michelson (Eds.), *Behavioral research methods in environmental design* (p. 337-360). New York: Van Nostrand Reinhold.

Lawton, M. P. (1986). *Environment and aging,* second edition. Albany, NY: Center for the Study of Aging.

Lawton, M. P. (1985). The elderly in context: Perspectives from environmental psychology and gerontology. *Environment and Behavior,* 17 (4), 501-519.

Lawton, M. P. (1981a). Alternative housing. *Journal of Gerontological Social Work,* 3 (3), 61-80.

Lawton, M. P. (1981b). Community supports for the aged. *Journal of Social Issues,* 37 (3), 102-115.

Lawton, M. P. (1978). Institutions and alternatives for older people. *Health and Social Work,* 3 (2), 108-134.

Lawton, M. P. (1970). Mortality, morbidity, and voluntary change of residence by older people. *Journal of the American Geriatrics Society,* 18 (10), 823-831.

Lawton, M. P., & Herzog, R. (1988). *Special research methods for gerontology: Society and Aging Series.* Amityville, NY: Baywood.

Lawton, M. P., Moss, M., Hoffman, C., Kleban, M., Ruckdeschel, K., & Winter, L. (2001). Valuation of life: A concept and a scale. *Journal of Aging and Health,* 13 (1), 3-31.

Lawton, M. P., Moss, M., Hoffman, C., Grant, R., Ten-Have, T., & Kleban, M. (1999). Health, valuation of life, and the wish to live. *Gerontologist,* 39 (4), 406-416.

Lawton, M. P., Moss, M., & Glicksman, A. (1990). Quality of the last year of life of older persons. *Milbank Quarterly,* 68 (1), 1-28.

Lawton, M. P., & Nahemow, L. (1973). Ecology and the aging process. In C. Eisdorfer & M. P. Lawton (Eds.), *Psychology of adult development and aging.* (pp. 619-674). Washington, D.C.: American Psychological Association.

Lawton, M. P., Newcomer, R., & Byerts, T. (Eds.) (1976). *Community planning for an aging society.* Stroudsburg, PA: Dowden, Hutchinson and Ross.

Moss, M., & Lawton, M. P. (1982). Time budgets of older people: A window on four lifestyles. *Journal of Gerontology,* 37 (1), 115-123.

Nahemow, L. (2000). The ecological theory of aging: Powell Lawton's legacy. In R. Rubinstein, M. Moss, & M. Kleban (Eds.), *The many dimensions of aging* (pp. 22-40). New York: Springer Publisher Company

Newcomer, R., & Griffin, C. (2000). Community planning and the elderly. In R. Rubinstein, M. Moss, & M. Kleban (Eds.), *The many dimensions of aging* (pp. 239-252). New York: Springer Publisher Company.

Newcomer, R., Lawton, M., & Byerts, T. (Eds.) (1986). *Housing an aging society.* New York: Van Nostrand Reinhold.

Rubinstein, R. & Parmalee, P. (1992). Attachment to place and the representation of the life course by the elderly. In I. Altman & S. Low (Eds.), *Place attachment* (pp. 139-165). New York: Plenum.

Scheidt, R. J. & Norris-Baker, C. (1999). Place therapies for older adults: Conceptual and interventive approaches. *International Journal of Aging and Human Development,* 48 (4), 1-15.

Powell Lawton's Contributions
to Long-Term Care Settings

Margaret P. Calkins

SUMMARY. The design of long-term care facilities has changed radically over the past three decades, due in large part to the pioneering work of Powell Lawton. His early conceptualizations of key principles for people with dementia–orientation, negotiability, personalization, social interaction and safety–were considered somewhat radical when first applied in the Weiss Institute. Now, several decades later, many of the design implications of these principles have been empirically validated, and are pervasive and considered standard practice in long-term care design. This paper traces the history of long-term care design over the past three decades, clearly demonstrating the influence of Powell Lawton's work. *[Article copies available for a fee from The Haworth Document Delivery Service: 1-800-HAWORTH. E-mail address: <getinfo@haworthpressinc.com> Website: <http://www.HaworthPress.com> © 2003 by The Haworth Press, Inc. All rights reserved.]*

KEYWORDS. Long-term care, design, built-environment, dementia, environment-behavior studies

Many of the readers of this article may have known Powell Lawton personally–some better than others. Those of us who knew him have our special

Margaret P. Calkins is President, I.D.E.A.S., Inc., 8055 Chardon Road, Kirtland, OH 44094.

[Haworth co-indexing entry note]: "Powell Lawton's Contributions to Long-Term Care Settings." Calkins, Margaret P. Co-published simultaneously in *Journal of Housing for the Elderly* (The Haworth Press, Inc.) Vol. 17, No. 1/2, 2003, pp. 67-84; and: *Physical Environments and Aging: Critical Contributions of M. Powell Lawton to Theory and Practice* (ed: Rick J. Scheidt, and Paul G. Windley) The Haworth Press, Inc., 2003, pp. 67-84. Single or multiple copies of this article are available for a fee from The Haworth Document Delivery Service [1-800-HAWORTH, 9:00 a.m. - 5:00 p.m. (EST). E-mail address: getinfo@haworthpressinc.com].

memories–of the first time we met him, of the times he would listen and engage in spirited discourse, or of the way he helped one think through a particularly challenging theorem. Powell had a special gift for reaching out and touching people–not just the hundreds of people he mentored, but even people he had only met once. It is, in part, his overriding concern for the individual–whether it be a person with dementia in a nursing home or a student in environmental psychology–that has contributed significantly to the impact he has had on long-term care.

LAWTON'S EARLY WORK

Thus, before exploring his impact on long-term care, it is important to start with a brief look at the context of his life. In 1947, he was about to head off to Oberlin College to study oboe, and, at the last minute, decided on Columbia University instead. Powell began his career at the Veterans Administration in Providence, RI, as Chief Clinical Psychologist. This was followed by 5 years at Norristown State Hospital, where he was Director of Clinical Training of psychologists and studied the psychological aspects of smoking.[1] In 1963, after several years of pursuing him, Arthur Waldman convinced Lawton to give up his smoking projects and join the Philadelphia Geriatric Center (PGC).

Powell transformed the Polisher Research Institute from a one-man office to a prodigious and incredibly prolific 60-person powerhouse. But as Elaine Brody points out in her foreword in *The Many Dimensions of Aging*, it is important to put the impact of this work in context:

> In 1963, no home for the aged included a research unit, and very few (if any) organizations of any kind had a research program focused on older people. The elderly and their families in the main were neglected, ignored, and in many ways oppressed by society . . . Social Security was just beginning to take hold. Medicare and Medicaid would not come into being until 1965, and Supplemental Security income did not exist until 1972. In those early 1960's, there was virtually no specialized housing for older people, nor were there long-term care services. (Brody, 2000, p. xvi)

In many ways, he came into this field at an auspicious moment, when the country was just beginning to realize that the growing number of elderly, both the healthy and independent, as well as those impaired by physical or cognitive deficits, had unique issues that needed to be addressed.

LAWTON'S MULTIFACETED CONTRIBUTIONS

Conceptualizing Environment-Behavior

His early work provided a number of conceptual frameworks that are still very useful today. I will not review his ecological theory (developed with Lucille Nahemow), his explorations of "the good life" (which we now call quality of life) or his stimulation and retreat theories, as most readers will be familiar with them. Part of their beauty is that they can be applied to the environment at a macro, policy-level scale as well as at the level of the micro environment. These theories and frameworks have shaped the thinking of many of today's scholars and will continue to influence tomorrow's scholars as well. For example, in 1977, he argued that:

> maintaining a marginally competent tenant in housing [senior housing with little or no service component] where the press level is too high will risk negative and maladaptive behavior. Sending such a person to a full nursing care institution may lower press excessively and cause negative and maladaptive behaviors. (Lawton, 1977, p. 10)

The solution he proposed was two-fold: create multi-level care campuses where people can reside in an environment that meets their competency levels, and create a level of care that is more supportive than that found in independent living situation but not as impoverished as most nursing home settings of the time. Thus, he argued early and persuasively for the development of what is now called assisted living, which provides adequate supports for moderately frail individuals.

Quality of Life

Beyond the theoretical frameworks he provided, at the crux of all of his work was his belief in and commitment to quality of life. No one else working at that time had his vision, dedication, and courage to pursue, as doggedly and as successfully, the prerequisites for achieving a high quality of life in old age. His work has bridged the substantial gulf that often exists between understanding and assessing an individual's situation and recognizing the necessity of developing planning principles and policies that positively affect elderly persons. He developed a battery of assessment instruments to help us understand that complex, multifaceted construct of quality of life and the various factors, both internal and external, which influence its expression. He was also a prolific writer and editor, disseminating this thinking to a huge audience—designers and providers as well as researchers concerned with long-term care. It is impossible to fully identify the ways in which these assessment instruments have impacted and changed the structure of long term care settings, but they have changed the way care is provided.

Applications to the Built Environment

Another unique aspect of Powell's work was its inclusion of the physical or built environment. At a time when few people were challenging how nursing homes were designed, he was instrumental in helping the Philadelphia Geriatric Center to build the Weiss Pavilion on a totally different set of assumptions. These assumptions were based on the needs of individuals compromised by cognitive impairment. Before most professionals gave this consideration, he began to conceptualize the critical dimensions of person-environment interactions for people with dementia, believing that defining such dimensions constitutes a necessary precursor to effective measurement. The basic principles he initially outlined included orientation, negotiability (autonomy in Activities of Daily Living or ADLs), personalization, social interaction and safety. To a great extent, these 5 principles have become the foundation for designing long-term care settings. A brief examination of 30 years of long-term care design will demonstrate his enormous influence on this field.

Before 1975, virtually all nursing homes were characterized by long, double-loaded corridors. These were usually dominated by a nursing station behind which staff could passively monitor residents' whereabouts and activities. Bedrooms were shared by two, four, or eight individuals. Unit size was almost always 60, as this number had been "determined" to maximize staffing efficiency. The one central day room was usually located across from the nursing station, and activity programs were virtually nonexistent (and hence did not require additional space).

Many of the basic assumptions about nursing home design and structure were challenged with the opening of the Weiss Pavilion at the Philadelphia Geriatric Center in 1978. The unit was designed for only 40 residents and the hallways were eliminated in favor of a large, open central space. This also maximized opportunities for residents to maintain orientation to the bedrooms (which were color coded), the nursing station (orange), the dining room (surrounded by a railing) and the other social spaces (e.g., gazebo). Lawton felt strongly that a sufficient number of individuals and opportunities for social contact were necessary to create a positive social milieu for these residents who experience so much difficulty in initiating activity and social contact.

The other significant contribution of the Weiss Pavilion was the post-occupancy evaluation that was conducted in the year after it opened, which added insight and depth to the hypotheses that the building represented. The results were encouraging, although not as dramatic as he had hoped.

> Performance on the indices of basic competence declined, as expected, but the more pliable behavioral variables did not decline, as one might expect them to on the basis of their initial correlations with basic competencies. Even more remarkably, in five instances improvement occurred, and in only one instance was there a significant decline. This pattern of findings, together with those from the behavior maps, confirms the pres-

ence of a clear prosthetic effect, to the point where the direction of decline was reversed in some instances to becoming improvement. (Lawton, Fulcomer, & Kleban, 1984, pp. 750-751)

Despite these positive results, the next decade saw little that was innovative in long term care design. Assisted living was beginning to be viewed as a viable option and alternative to nursing level care. Nursing homes, however, continued to be built with long corridors, no orientation cues, and limited attention to social spaces. But the seeds were sown, and just took longer to come to fruition. The late 1980s saw several projects that drew upon the work of the Weiss Institute, along with Powell's other ongoing research.

The Corinne Dolan Alzheimer Center [CDAC] at Heather Hill Hospital, Health and Care Center, was the first of the "next generation" projects for people with dementia. It followed and further refined many of the same basic principles as the Weiss Institute. It had a similar open plan, although the scale was substantially smaller, with 12 residents on each of two pods. The open plan provided a high degree of visibility of the bedroom entrances to help maintain residents' orientation. This was further enhanced by the presence of a large, well-lit display case at each entrance, filled with personal mementoes of each resident. Negotiability, or autonomy in ADLs, was addressed by creating highly visible toilet areas in each bedroom, specially modified closets to support independence in dressing, and access to a kitchen to permit continuation of familiar self-supporting skills in normal everyday living conditions (as opposed to restricted institutional living conditions). Residents furnished their own bedrooms, including all of their own furniture to enhance their sense of personal space and privacy. Social interaction was supported through the availability of a number of different spaces, several with very different character, in which a rich and varied program of activities was offered. Finally, security was handled in a discrete manner, allowing residents unrestricted access to an adjacent two-acre secure courtyard through wide glass doors. The doors that led to the parking lot, however, were dark and windowless, to limit their appeal.

Immediately following the opening of CDAC, Woodside Place opened in Oakmont, PA. This facility took a slightly different approach, although the differences are in the details, not in the underlying principles which Powell had articulated. Rather than an open plan, each 12-person household consisted of a short corridor, with the kitchen and dining room at one end, and a door that led to the courtyard at the other end. Each household was identified with a color and a theme, expressed in a quilt that hung in each dining room. Bedroom entrances had a place for residents to display a photo or two, either a current image of the residents or meaningful images from their past. Residents had similar levels of access to the kitchen to enhance continuity with familiar daily routines. The spine of the building, which served to connect the three households, the offices and several other program spaces, became a successful component of the social life of the residents, who would stroll along this connecting corridor, passing and greeting other individuals taking a walk (Danes, 2002).

There are several aspects to these projects that make them direct descendents of Powell Lawton's work at the Philadelphia Geriatric Center. First, both projects carried forward Lawton's belief that a smaller scale was important. He actually expressed some concerns that groupings of 12 residents might be too small, but felt it made a good experiment to contrast with the 40-bed Weiss Institute (Lawton, 1988). Both projects also engaged in rigorous post-occupancy research. The research at Woodside Place followed the same basic structure as the PGC evaluation, evaluating global outcomes of the complete environment. The CDAC research, conversely, undertook a series of eight individualized, controlled studies of single environmental elements to explore the impact of single features of the environment. It is worth noting that both were assisted living–not nursing home–projects.

Both these projects received significant attention through conference presentations and numerous publications, and served to spur other organizations to explore strategies to respond to the set of basic principles Powell Lawton developed. A number of these principles have become common practice in long-term care design. Their efficacy is also being borne out by research. The rest of this paper focuses on the expression and evaluation, where available, of Powell Lawton's principles for the design of care settings for people with dementia.

LAWTON'S PRINCIPLES FOR THE DESIGN OF CARE SETTINGS

Setting Size

Although not generally included as a discrete principle, Lawton was concerned about the size of care units, because it is related to density, which affects stimulation levels. As mentioned above, the Weiss Pavilion broke with tradition by creating a distinct setting for 40 residents (instead of 60), while the CDAC and Woodside Place were based on multiples of 12 person households. In a review of research on dementia care settings, Day and Calkins (in press) identify several studies which suggest that "smaller units (less than 20 residents) are associated with less anxiety and depression; less usage of antibiotics and psychotropic drugs; higher motor functions; more mobility, social interaction, and friendship formation; and more supervision and interaction between staff and residents" (see Annerstedt, 1993, 1994; McAllister & Silverman, 1999; McCracken & Fitzwater, 1989; Moore, 1999; Netten, 1993; Skea & Lindsay, 1996). In terms of design, the trend in construction is for smaller units. An analysis of facility plans published in several long-term care trade journals over the past 20 years indicates that the average unit size has decreased from 30 in the 1980s to 19 beds in the 1990s.[2]

Orientation

Recognizing that people with dementia find it harder to rely on their memories to orient themselves within a space and to find desired locations, the Weiss Pavilion was designed to enhance the resident's ability to have direct visibility to desired locations (bedrooms, nursing station, dining room and shared social spaces). This principle has been taken seriously by designers, and the vast majority of dementia care settings that are constructed today recognize the value of maximizing orientation (see Illustration 1).

The two most common approaches include an open plan, where the bedrooms open directly onto the main shared social spaces, and cluster plans, where the bedrooms are arrayed along short corridors that lead to the shared social spaces (see Illustration 2).

Beyond unit layout, organizations also recognize the importance of supporting orientation to various locations–particularly the bedroom. The Weiss Pavilion color-coded each bedroom entrance to help residents find their own bedroom, while CDAC provided enclosed display cases at the bedroom entrance and Woodside Place provided a place to display a few photographs. Research has shown that personalized cues at the bedroom entrance can increase independence in locating the bedroom (Namazi, Rosner, & Rechlin, 1991; Nolan, Mathews, Truesdell-Todd & VanDorp, 2002). The prevalence in most dementia facilities of some form of personalized display at the bedroom entrance (c.f., Anders, 1994; Best Practices, 1997; Cohen & Day, 1993; Kromm & Kromm, 1985; Tames, 1992; Tetlow, 1995) indicates the widespread acceptance of the value of this principle.

Negotiability

For Lawton, negotiability related to the ability to continue to engage in and successfully complete basic activities of daily living and maintain functional independence. There has been less consistency in design solutions that address negotiability. Bathing has received substantial attention in the literature over the past several years, and while there have been some advances in the design of tubs which do not require residents to be strapped to a chair and hoisted over

ILLUSTRATION 1. Bridges Medical Services, Designed by Horty Elving

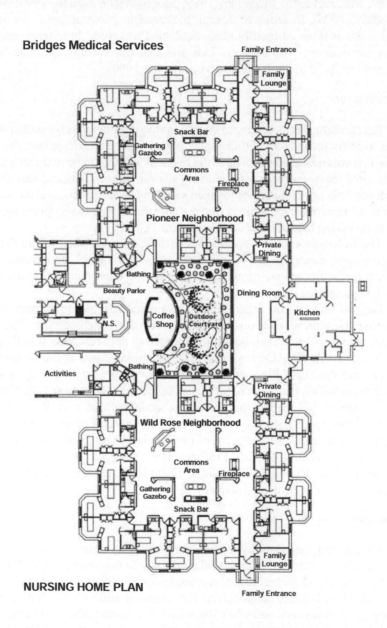

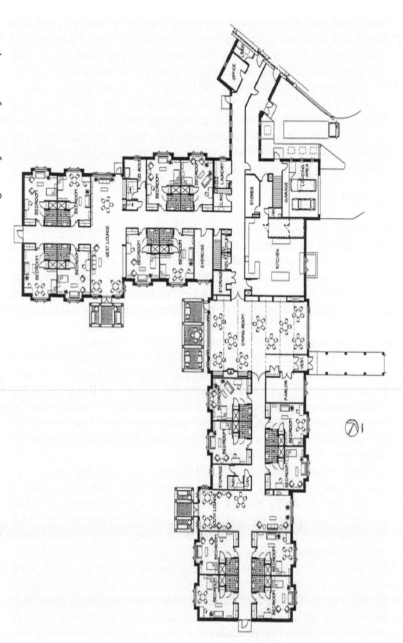

ILLUSTRATION 2. Helen D. Schubert Villa, Notre Dame, IN, Designed by The Troyer Group

the top of a tub, the design of tub *rooms* is still driven by institutional sanitation standards, and does not generally support resident independence. Similarly, while there is convincing evidence that the type of grab bars specified by the Americans with Disabilities Act are not supportive of the toilet transfer needs of frail older individuals (Sanford, 2001), and that appropriate alternatives do exist (Sanford & Malassigne, 1999; Sanford, 2002), few facilities incorporate these more supportive features. Nor has there been much attention to developing environmental support for independent dressing, although one furniture manufacturer has a closet that can have one section available to the residents while the other sections are secured.

Personalization

At the time the Weiss Pavilion was built, nursing homes were viewed primarily as clinical care settings. But with the increase in the number of people with dementia, who often did not need sophisticated clinical care but rather a safe and supportive setting in which to live (often for a number of years), the emphasis began to change from being a *nursing* home to a nursing *home* (Day & Calkins, in press). Until recently, nursing homes routinely provided all the furniture and equipment for residents, who were allowed to bring in clothes and possibly a few knick-knacks to "personalize" their rooms.

Although it is still common for nursing homes to provide all the residents' furniture, there is a general trend toward allowing residents to bring more personal belongings with them when they move. In assisted living facilities, residents are often encouraged to provide most, if not all, of the furniture in their bedrooms or apartments. These belongings are seen as a reflection of the individuals' identities–who they are, what they accomplished, and what was important to them in their lifetimes.

In addition to personal items for their bedrooms, facilities are also increasingly recognizing the need to replicate, to the greatest extent possible, the familiar daily routines and activities residents engaged in when they lived in the community. Thus, spaces are designed increasingly to reflect not the hospital day room, but the living room or den of the homes of the people who now live there (see Illustration 3).

Also, an increasing percentage of facilities are including a kitchen on their dementia care units, although how the kitchen is used is highly variable (Marsden, Meehan & Calkins, 2001). Overall, Day and Calkins (in press) note that non-institutional environments characterized as having homelike or enhanced ambiance are associated with a number of positive outcomes, including: improved intellectual and emotional well-being, enhanced social interaction, reduced agitation/aggression, reduced trespassing and exit-seeking, greater preference and

ILLUSTRATION 3. Harbour House, Greendale, WI, Designed by KM Development Corp.

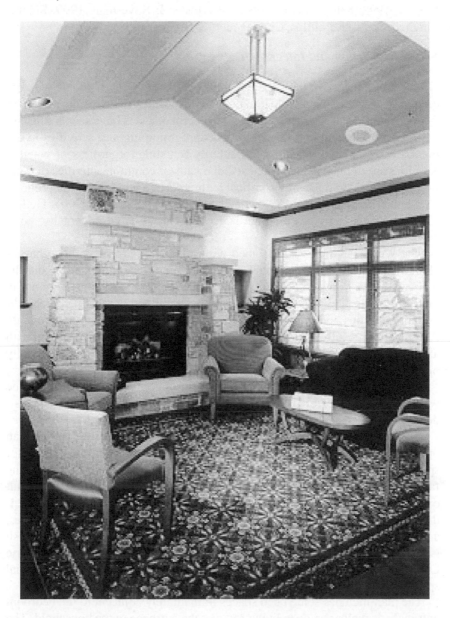

pleasure, improved functionality and motor functioning, lower usage of tranquilizing drugs, and less anxiety (see Annerstedt, 1994; Cohen-Mansfield & Werner, 1998; Kihlgren et al., 1992; McAllister & Silverman, 1999; Sloane, Mitchell, Preisser, Phillips, Commander, & Burker, 1998).

Social Interaction and Integration

One consequence of the impaired cognitive functioning of people with dementia is a decreased ability to initiate activities, which often results in a lower frequency of social interaction. The past several decades have seen a substantial increase in attention directed towards programming and activities in dementia care settings. Indeed, a full activity schedule (regardless of whether activities are defined as structured social events or common activities of daily living) is considered one of the critical hallmarks of a good dementia program (Alzheimer's Association, 1997; Bowlby, 1993; Calkins, 1988, 2001; Hellen, 1998). How the activities program is accommodated environmentally, however, is quite varied.

The Weiss Pavilion was designed with a large, central open area that included the dining room and main activity areas, the nursing station and the hallway directly outside resident bedrooms. Whenever residents were not in their bedrooms, they were in areas where the likelihood of meeting other individuals, and thus opportunities for spontaneous social interaction, were high. A number of recently constructed projects follow this same basic pattern, with all of the shared social spaces of the unit clustered together and essentially open to each other (see Illustration 4).

This allows residents to easily preview an ongoing activity to determine whether they want to join it. However, it can also make it difficult to keep residents focused on an activity, as there are many distractions.

An alternative approach was pioneered at the CDAC, which combined an open plan with a number of discrete activity rooms. This allowed both for spontaneous interaction and greetings of people casually walking around the facility, with more focused and intense social interaction occurring as a result of structured programs. By separating the program spaces, it was felt that residents would be less distracted and better able to concentrate on the activities, and people, before them. The Madlyn & Leonard Abramson Center for Jewish Living (which is the new replacement facility for the Philadelphia Geriatric Center) reflects this "layered" type of plan, which mixes both open social spaces with some more private, enclosed spaces (Illustration 5).

The plan includes some open spaces immediately adjacent to the bedroom entrances as well as an open living room at the entrance to the household. The

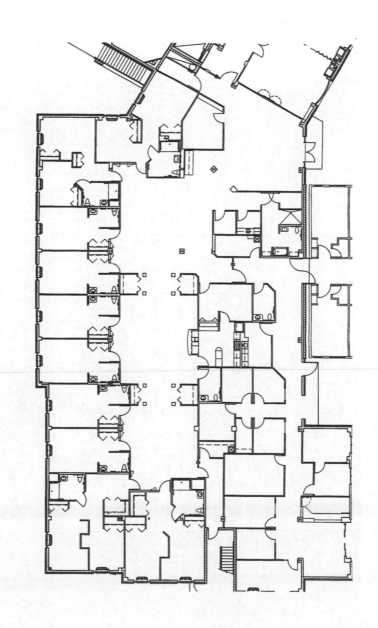

ILLUSTRATION 4. Friendship Village of Columbus, Columbus, OH, Designed by Maddox NBD

ILLUSTRATION 5. Madlyn & Leonard Abramson Center for Jewish Living, Philadelphia, PA, Designed by Ewing Cole Cherry Brott/Nelson Tremaine Partnership

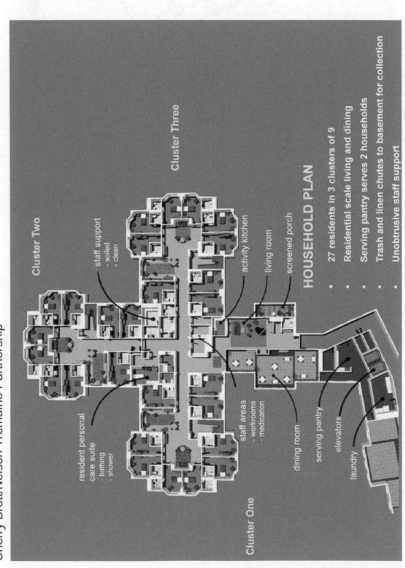

Cluster Two

Cluster Three

Cluster One

staff support
- soiled
- clean

activity kitchen

living room

screened porch

resident personal
care suite
- bathing
- shower

staff areas
- workrooms
- medication

dining room

serving pantry

elevators

laundry

HOUSEHOLD PLAN

- 27 residents in 3 clusters of 9
- Residential scale living and dining
- Serving pantry serves 2 households
- Trash and linen chutes to basement for collection
- Unobtrusive staff support

dining room is enclosed, and there are small rooms adjacent to the dining room that can be used for small group meals or other group activities.

Safety

The cognitive impairments associated with dementia, as well as more general age-related physical deficits, can threaten the safety and security of people with Alzheimer's disease and those who provide care for them. Too often safety is simply interpreted as creating a secured unit so residents cannot wander away. Yet the issue of safety is more complex than simply managing egress control. The cognitively-impaired individual may not be able to understand the potential hazards in any given situation, and thus needs to be able to be closely monitored by staff, ideally in an unobtrusive manner.

The Weiss Pavilion, with its open floor plan, provided the ideal design for the monitoring of residents by staff. The centrally located nursing station had clear and uninterrupted visibility of virtually all resident care areas. This design also enabled residents to easily find staff, which can enhance their sense of security, or their own *perceived* safety. However, changes in both philosophy and reimbursement in long-term care over the past decade have altered the way nursing stations are designed and used. Reduced staffing levels have significantly decreased the amount of time staff spend sitting behind the nursing station. Instead, staff are "on the floor" giving care to the residents. The nursing station is also viewed as a vestige of the old medical philosophy–settings that are trying to feel more residential often eliminate the nursing station completely. Yet being able to easily, and ideally unobtrusively, monitor residents is still a critical issue. Not surprisingly, most of the open plans provide staff greater visibility of the residents than do many of the cluster plans (compare, for instance, the open plan shown in Illustration 4 with the cluster plan of Illustration 2).

There have been a number of technological advances that can make it easier to monitor residents unobtrusively, identifying when they cross a threshold, or exceed a certain distance from a central monitor. Increasingly, these technologies make use of silent staff pagers, which helps to minimize the level of meaningless, noxious noise in the environment (from call bells or other alarms that are not answered promptly). It is often a challenge, however, to get state regulators to allow these newer technologies. There are also products such as lights that turn on slowly to allow for the older eye to adjust gradually as the light level increases, bed and chair alarms that alert staff when a resident who is at risk of falling is trying to rise, and timers which turn appliances on and off automatically. Because these can be incorporated in virtually any environment, they will not be reviewed in detail here.

FURTHER REFLECTIONS

The preceding illustrations provide substantial evidence that the basic principles developed by Powell Lawton in the early 1970s for creating successful dementia care settings have been both borne out by research and accepted by care providers. What is interesting to note about some of these projects, and many others not featured here, is that they are no longer solely for people with dementia. While the 1980s and early 1990s sought to define what was "special" about special care units for people with dementia, the past several years have seen a cross-over of design principles that were once considered "dementia-specific" to being considered appropriate for other individuals with more physical, rather than cognitive impairments. This shift may reflect a growing understanding that people with dementia are *people* first, and we must consider their needs as individuals first, as older individuals second, and only then as older people with dementia. Thus, principles that support people with dementia are also likely to be supportive of people without dementia.

It is hard to summarize in this limited space the myriad contributions Powell Lawton had on long term care. Much like the discovery of electricity, which has touched all our lives despite our not knowing Benjamin Franklin, Powell's work has touched, in one way or another, directly or indirectly, the lives of virtually every older person in the country. It will continue to do so for decades to come.

NOTES

1. Just think how different national trends in smoking might be now if he had dedicated his significant talent to *that* field!
2. Sources of descriptions of actual facilities included *Nursing Homes Magazine* (1972-present), *Long Term Care Administrator* (1983 to present), *Provider* (1987 to present) and *Assisted Living Today* (1993 to present). Additional sources include results of several national competitions ("Design for Aging" sponsored by the American Institute of Architects, and several competitions sponsored by the above-mentioned trade journals) and design guide books for dementia care facilities.

REFERENCES

Alzheimer's Association. (1997). *Key elements of dementia care.* Chicago, IL: Author. 67-80.
Anders, K. T. (1994). Special care. *Contemporary Long Term Care, 17*(2), 48-49.
Annerstedt, L. (1993). Development and consequences of group living in Sweden. *Social Science and Medicine, 37*(12), 1529-1538.

Annerstedt, L. (1994). An attempt to determine the impact of group living care in comparison to traditional long-term care on demented elderly patients. *Aging Clinical Experimental Research*, 6(5), 372-380.

Best Practices. (1997). *Contemporary Long Term Care*, 20(8), 48-49.

Bowlby, C. (1993). *Therapeutic activities for persons disabled by Alzheimer's disease and related disorders*. Baltimore: Aspen Publishers.

Brody, E. (2000). Foreword. In Rubenstein, R., Moss, M., & Kleban, M. (Eds.), *The many dimensions of aging*. New York: Springer Publishing Company.

Calkins, M. P. (1988). *Design for dementia: Planning environments for the elderly and the confused*. Owings Mills: National Health Publishing.

Calkins, M. P. (2001). *Creating successful dementia care settings*. Baltimore: Health Professions Press.

Cohen, U., & Day, K. (1993). *Contemporary environments for people with dementia*. Baltimore, MD: Johns Hopkins University Press.

Cohen-Mansfield, J., & Werner, P. (1998). The effects of an enhanced environment on nursing home residents who pace. *The Gerontologist*, 38(2), 199-208.

Danes, S. (2002). Creating an environment for community. *Alzheimer's Care Quarterly*, 3(1), 66-71.

Day K., & Calkins, M. P. (in press). Design and Dementia. In R. Bechtel (Ed), *Handbook for Environmental Psychology*. John Wiley & Sons.

Hellen, C. (1998). *Alzheimer's disease: Activity focused care*. Woburn, MA: Butterworth Heinemann.

Kihlgren, M., Bråne, G., Karlsson, I., Kuremyr, D., Leissner, P., & Norberg, A. (1992). Long-term influences on demented patients in different caring milieus, a collective living unit and a nursing home: A descriptive study. *Dementia*, 3, 342-349.

Kromm, D., & Kromm, Y. H. N. (1985). A nursing unit designed for Alzheimer's Disease patients at Newton Presbyterian Manor. *Nursing Homes*, 34(3), 30-31.

Lawton, M. P. (1977). An ecological theory of aging applied to elderly housing. *JAE 31(1), 8-10.*

Lawton, M. P. (1988). Personal communication with author.

Lawton, M. P., Fulcomer, M. & Kleban, M. (1984). Architecture for the mentally impaired. *Environment and Behavior*, 16(6), 730-757.

Marsden, J., Meehan, R., & Calkins, M. (2001). Therapeutic kitchens for residents with dementia. *American Journal of Alzheimer's Disease and Other Dementias*, 16(5); 303-312.

McAllister, C. L., & Silverman, M. A. (1999). Community formation and community roles among persons with Alzheimer's disease: A comparative study of experiences in a residential Alzheimer's facility and a traditional nursing home. *Qualitative Health Research*, 9(1), 65-85.

McAllister, C. L., & Silverman, M. A. (1999). Community formation and community roles among persons with Alzheimer's disease: A comparative study of experiences in a residential Alzheimer's facility and a traditional nursing home. *Qualitative Health Research*, 9(1), 65-85.

McCracken, A. L., & Fitzwater, E. (1989). The right environment for Alzheimer's: Which is better–open versus closed units? Here's how to tailor the answer to the patient. *Geriatric Nursing*, 10(6), 293-294.

Moore, K. D. (1999). Dissonance in the dining room: A study of social interaction in a special care unit. *Qualitative Health Research, 9*(1), 133-155.

Namazi, K. H., Rosner, T. T., & Rechlin, L. (1991). Long-term memory cuing to reduce visuo-spatial disorientation in Alzheimer's disease patients in a special care unit. *American Journal of Alzheimer's Care and Related Disorders and Research, 6*(6), 10-15.

Netten, A. (1993). *A positive environment? Physical and social influences on people with senile dementia in residential care.* Aldershot, England: Ashgate.

Nolan, B., Mathews, M., Truesdell-Todd, G. & VanDorp, A. (2002). Evaluation of the effect of orientation cues on wayfinding in persons with dementia. *Alzheimer's Care Quarterly, 3*(1), 47-49.

Sanford, J. (2001). *Access to toilet and bathing facilities.* Washington, DC: US Access Board; 2001, Final Report.

Sanford, J. (2002). Time to get rid of those old gray grab bars and get yourself a shiney new pair. *Alzheimer's Care Quarterly, 3*(1): 25-31.

Sanford, J., & Malassigne, P. (1999). An E for ADAAG: The case for ADA Accessibility Guidelines for the elderly based on three studies of toilet transfer. *Physical & Occupational Therapy in Geriatrics, 16*(3/4): 39-58.

Skea, D., & Lindesay, J. (1996). An evaluation of two models of long-term residential care for elderly people with dementia. *International Journal of Geriatric Psychiatry, 11*, 233-241.

Sloane, P. D., Mitchell, C. M., Preisser, J. S., Phillips, C., Commander, C., & Burker, E. (1998). Environmental correlates of resident agitation in Alzheimer's disease special care units. *Journal of the American Geriatrics Society, 46*(7), 862-869.

Tames, S. (1992). Designing with residents in mind. *Provider, 18*(7), 17-28.

Tetlow, K. (1995). Exercise by design. *Contemporary Long Term Care, 18*(3), 38-42.

Quality of Life
and Place-Therapy

Habib Chaudhury

SUMMARY. The multidimensional "quality of life" conceptual model is one of Powell Lawton's landmark contributions in gerontology that has influenced several studies, including the exploratory study of "place-therapy." Key dimensions of the QOL model, such as temporality, subjectivity influenced and inspired this study that explored reminiscence of personally meaningful past places among cognitively intact and impaired residents in four nursing homes. The therapeutic potential of place-based reminiscence is proposed as an avenue in understanding and enhancing the quality of life for older adults in long-term care facilities. Place is used a means to recollect the rich narrative of lived experiences of the individuals who often become anonymous care-receiving nursing home "residents." Potential avenues for further inquiry in place-therapy are indicated. *[Article copies available for a fee from The Haworth Document Delivery Service: 1-800-HAWORTH. E-mail address: <getinfo@haworthpressinc.com> Website: <http://www.HaworthPress.com> © 2003 by The Haworth Press, Inc. All rights reserved.]*

KEYWORDS. Quality of life, place, dementia, reminiscence, long-term care, therapy, well-being

Habib Chaudhury is affiliated with Simon Fraser University.

The author expresses gratitude to Professor Gerald Weisman at the University of Wisconsin-Milwaukee for his guidance in the exploratory study on place-based recollection.

[Haworth co-indexing entry note]: "Quality of Life and Place-Therapy." Chaudhury, Habib. Co-published simultaneously in *Journal of Housing for the Elderly* (The Haworth Press, Inc.) Vol. 17, No. 1/2, 2003, pp. 85-103; and: *Physical Environments and Aging: Critical Contributions of M. Powell Lawton to Theory and Practice* (ed: Rick J. Scheidt, and Paul G. Windley) The Haworth Press, Inc., 2003, pp. 85-103. Single or multiple copies of this article are available for a fee from The Haworth Document Delivery Service [1-800-HAWORTH, 9:00 a.m. - 5:00 p.m. (EST). E-mail address: getinfo@haworthpressinc.com].

(A PERSONAL) INTRODUCTION

The young gerontologist should be especially attuned to her or his own personality style and seek matches for these in choices made at various stages of their careers. (Lawton, 2000, pp. 195-196)

Among all the qualities that various researchers and scholars have mentioned to describe the contribution of Powell Lawton, the one that stands out most distinctly for me is–Powell Lawton as an educator. My first contact with Powell Lawton was at a workshop in the School of Architecture and Urban Planning at the University of Wisconsin-Milwaukee in mid-1990s. He was participating in the event along with other researchers in aging and environment. For me, a doctoral student, meeting Powell Lawton in person was obviously a privilege and honor as I was beginning to appreciate the depth and breadth of his work's influence in gerontology. However, beyond witnessing first hand the depth of his insights in aging and environment issues and his unique humane approach, I was struck by his interest in my work and his sharing of views in that regard. As I mentioned to him my research focus on place experience and the potential of recollection of past places as a therapeutic activity for older adults, he shared with me how he had discovered the importance of place in older adults in his numerous studies. He mentioned to me that in many of his interactions with the elderly, place-related experiences had come up spontaneously and frequently. In my brief discussion with him on that occasion, Powell stressed the centrality of place in people's lives, especially in later years, and suggested the term "place-therapy" that immediately captured my aspirations in that area.

Subsequently, on a number of other occasions, I had the opportunity to talk with Powell Lawton and seek his thoughts and suggestions on this exploratory area of place-therapy. He considered this area of research as worthwhile, especially in the context of people with dementia. Powell believed that research in dementia care should explore more direct interaction with the person with dementia and he was very encouraging to me in pursuing this avenue of research of place-based reminiscence work with residents with dementia. He was very supportive in exploring innovative ways of developing activities that could be meaningful for persons with cognitive impairment, and was generous in sharing his viewpoints on place-oriented recollection. Powell's multidimensional view of "quality of life" influenced my thinking at looking at place-based reminiscence from a holistic approach and shaped my understanding of the therapeutic potential of using personally meaningful past places as themes for conducting reminiscence sessions. In this paper, I will outline the key aspects of the theoretical framework of "quality of life" as they relate to the exploratory work in "place-therapy" with some case illustrations, and suggest some avenues for further exploration in this line of inquiry.

LONG-TERM CARE FACILITY AND POTENTIAL OF PLACE-BASED REMINISCENCE

A definition of quality of life may be offered here: Quality of life is the multi-dimensional evaluation, by both intrapersonal and social-normative criteria, of the person-environment system of an individual in time past, current, and anticipated. (Lawton, 1991, p. 6)

In a series of my own research findings, there has been a strong tendency for positive emotional states to occur in older people who are more engaged with other people, leisure activities, and their environments. One of my current ideological missions is to promote the idea that a neglected route to positive mental health for older people is to find ways of enhancing such engagement. A much more difficult idea for research is whether there are other extroverted means by which people can enhance their engagement with their own goals, thoughts, or memories . . . *ways of making one's interiority more novel, challenging, and appealing, as perhaps in self-guided reminiscence, is a task for future clinician.* [italics added] (Lawton, 2000, pp. 192-193)

The fundamental premise of Powell Lawton's (1991) conceptualization of "quality of life" is recognition of the breadth and depth of older adults' lives and the inherent meanings. This conceptual model appreciates the complexity of the concept and provides a systemic approach in understanding the person, as well as emphasizes the importance of socio-psychological aspects in life beyond the traditional approaches that look at decrements from a baseline. Lawton's (1991) quality of life conceptualization proposes four evaluative sectors of "good life": psychological well-being, perceived quality of life, behavioral competence and objective environment. At the core of these four sectors is "self" as the integrating reality of individuals. For example, quality of life gains added dimensions in the long-term care setting as older adults become part of and subject to organizational policies, care philosophies and regulations. Issues of personal choice, interaction with staff members, dependence, self-esteem, etc., have a profound significance because for many people this will be their "residence" for the balance of their lives.

To the extent long-term care is based on institutional values, policies, and procedures, residents face the potential of losing their self-identity. Nursing homes are places that stand in contrast with community living where "to-be-residents" have lived all of their lives. The facilities symbolize withdrawal from community and institutionalization of physical dependency. There is limited opportunity for self-expression in the nursing home where the organizational and collective approaches of caregiving quite often dominate the social and physical environment. Self-identity and personal meaning are largely over-taken by institutional policies and routines (Rubinstein & Parmelee, 1992).

In order to be truthful to the objective of ensuring quality of care, it is critical to gain an understanding of the subjective meaning of quality of life for the residents. The four sectors of Lawton's quality of life conceptualization: behavioral competence, psychological well-being, perceived quality of life, and the objective environment interrelate to give form and shape to behavior, environment and experience. To create a meaningful living environment in the nursing home, it is critical that we understand these several sectors, not in isolation, but in an integrative fashion that resembles real life experience for the residents. This process of understanding should begin in grasping the unique identities of the residents reflected through their personal pasts. Part of this subjective understanding is to recognize and appreciate the residents' life histories—who are they as individuals? What are their values, preferences, beliefs, and attitudes? What is the nature and meaning of homes that have been an important part of their lives? What are the life experiences associated with those places?

For the institutionalized older person, reminiscence of significant places from the past could be a powerful means of remembering one's life course. This may be particularly salient for people with dementia who have difficulties in maintaining their sense of selves in the face of the continuing erosion of identity associated with this progressing disease. The potential contribution of reminiscence may be substantial (Gibson, 1994) by capitalizing on what can be remembered from the distant past to help counter this threat to personhood. Moreover, personal memories may be somewhat more accessible than non-personal events, e.g., memories of the particular home where the resident raised her children over several years may be relatively easier to recall than the name of the president of the United States at a certain time in the past (Woods & McKiernan, 1995).

The transition to a nursing home symbolizes not only loss of a familiar environment, but, in many instances, also separation from the home with which one has strong emotional attachment. Moreover, the majority of long-term care facilities are "nonplaces" that afford few links with one's personal or cultural past. The typical care setting, both in its social and physical aspects, reflects institutional policies and procedures as opposed to the personally meaningful place the resident has left behind. Facilities designed on the medical model of care promote adoption of generalized social roles such as "old" and "sick" (Piper & Langer, 1986) and deprive individuals of their familiar and meaningful environmental past.

There is evidence that reminiscence sessions with institutionalized people with dementia can be therapeutic (Woods & McKiernan, 1995). However, this research remains mostly in the domain of the procedural aspects, i.e., guidelines and techniques for conducting reminiscence sessions, with little attention given to the potential of substantive themes for reminiscence. Major efforts have been made regarding the "mechanism" of reminiscence sessions with the focus placed on their structure, processes, and application in the care of older people; little effort has been directed toward the content, themes, and meaning of reminiscence. There has not been any study looking at the probable variation in recollection across different topics of reminiscence. Although there is anecdotal support that experience of place "creeps into" recollections (Gibson, 1994), the potential of using place as an explicit reminiscence theme remains unexplored. Within the context of an unfamiliar nursing home environment, remembering significant past places presents a promising therapeutic process and may make life in an institution a little more bearable for its cognitively impaired residents. Remembering the personal past may provide the continuity that is personally meaningful for the residents. Within the unfamiliar social-physical environment of a nursing home, recalling past events, activities and places may provide psychological support to one's sense of self worth.

Second, remembrance of past places can help in redefining aspects of the self in the current changed environmental context. The construction of the past could be seen as a "psychological action, not just passive mirroring" (Rosenmayr, 1982). Beyond the nostalgic recollection of the past, guided reminiscence sessions can be a consciously engaging process for the older adult. This process can be mindful and dynamic as new aspects are brought in, familiar experiences are reinterpreted in a fresh light and in this process the self is *rediscovered*. The prospect of rediscovering the self is particularly intriguing for people with dementia. As the sense of self seems to gradually erode in the conditions of dementia, recollection of personal past offers the person a potential avenue for preservation and re-construction of the self-identity within the different life circumstances. Although there is a conceptual recognition of the potential of reminiscence as a reconstructive process for self-identity in older adults (Kitwood, 1997)–and places as a contributing factor in the process of evolving self (Gibson, 1994)–there has not been any empirical study exploring these issues in older adults with dementia. Also, the potential influence of a nursing home environment on stimulating (or lack thereof) residents' environmental memories need to be acknowledged. Presence of various aspects of the long-term care setting, environmental or psychosocial, can help reconnect with the past. For example, a resident's opportunity of walking in a garden in a nursing home may trigger her memories of gardening at her home. On the other hand, a resident who had lived all along in urban locations may not be environmentally stimulated in a rural nursing home context.

EXPLORING "PLACE-THERAPY"

The exploratory study in place-therapy reported here (Chaudhury, in press, 1999) is based on the inescapable premise that human experience occurs within the context of place. Places, especially personally meaningful ones, may serve as mnemonic anchors in autobiographical recollections, even for the cognitively impaired, and be a means of recalling who we are. A conceptual framework with recollection of past places as an ongoing dialogue between "I" and "Me," based on James' (1892) and Mead's (1934) theoretical approach of "self" guided the empirical study. The study explored, among others, the following interrelated research questions:

a. What are the emergent themes in recollection of past places for cognitively intact residents in long-term care settings?
b. Is place recollected by cognitively impaired residents?
c. What are the dimensions of place recollection by cognitively impaired residents?
d. Can place-related prompts trigger recollection of past places by cognitively impaired residents?

The study draws on interviews with eight cognitively intact residents, fifteen family members of residents with dementia, and thirteen residents with dementia. All residents were living in four nursing homes in Milwaukee, Wisconsin. Generic questions exploring past places, e.g., homes, neighborhoods, schools, etc., were used in interviews with cognitively intact residents and family members. Place-related biographical information and personal and generic photographs (based on interviews with residents' family members) were used as prompts in conversations with cognitively impaired residents.

Several themes emerged from the interviews and conversations with cognitively intact and impaired individuals. While the substantive themes were of interest for the cognitively intact group, the question was much more fundamental for people with dementia: can people with dementia recall places from their personal past? The study provides support for an affirmative response to this exploratory question. Residents with dementia could recollect segments and episodes of their past places, especially childhood places, when prompted by personally meaningful facts that served as triggers in retrieving these memories. More important, the places recollected acted as vehicles for remembering various life events and experiences. Personal photographs were especially valuable in this process of remembering the past (Chaudhury, in press). The diversity of emerging themes points out the complexity and interconnected nature of places in the narrative of life–and how one's identity is grounded in them.

For the people whose place-stories are the foundation of this study, past places are not a collection of empty spaces or mere objective locations, nor a realm of pure subjective perspective–but a middle ground (see Weisman, Chaudhury & Moore, 2000). Places are personal worlds anchored in physical reality through personally meaningful events, activities, and experiences. These meanings are held together with the subjective perceptions, preferences, and emotions of the individuals. The multifaceted nature of place in life experience points out the richness with which it allows us to understand lives and the individuals who lived them.

The centrality of home in one's life experience, as evidenced in previous studies, is also supported in this study for both groups of residents. The subjective aspects of these home-related memories make them especially potent in continuation of the sense of self over time. They provide the symbolic lifeline in the natural need for sustaining self-identity. The success of using individual residents' home-related photographs and narrative information to trigger memories in this study validates the significance of these artifacts in the residents' lives. In "medicalization" of the caregiving process in a nursing home, the sense of uniqueness of the self-identity can be maintained with the creative use of these memorabilia. In particular, in the sea of psychological, social, and environmental changes for a resident with dementia, these elements of the past can act as an anchor–the chain that connects things in their fragmented world.

TEMPORALITY

The temporal aspect of quality of life emphasizes the dynamic, ongoing nature of the person-environment system. Specifically, remembered qualities of the past are present in the frames of reference by which qualities of the present and future are evaluated. For their own sake, qualities of the past remain active as memories and reminiscences. (Lawton, 1991, p. 7)

One central theme in Lawton's quality of life conceptual model is the recognition and significance of temporal context. Lawton emphasized the dynamic nature of person-environment interaction through, among other aspects, the dimension of time in shaping one's evaluation, preference and attitudes in the current environment. This reality of temporal impact on a person's socio-environmental interaction is particularly salient in the act of recollection. The process of remembering the past is an activity distinctly imbued with temporal depth. It is *now* that we remember about *then*. Recollection of events and places from the past in the present is based upon our understanding and experience of the world in a linear sequence. I cannot "be" now and "be" then at the same time. Given this physical-temporal reality, the mental act of recollection creates a bridge between temporal planes. In some instances, when the recollection is vivid and emotionally charged, the apparent boundary between past and present becomes permeable and plastic.

Personally significant places provide a means to structure and store meaning of our pasts. But in conscious remembrance of the places, we not only create a link between now and then, but we also serve the more pragmatic concern of venturing forth into the future. Memories provide grounding for expectation and form a sense of continuity. Remembering the past is primarily a nostalgic endeavor, but it is also a process of recovery and reclamation. In remembering our past experiences, we rediscover our own nature and in the process expand our understanding of ourselves. A mirror helps us to look at ourselves and focus our attention on our physical attributes, and in that process we become more cognizant of our bodily appearance. Remembering allows us that same view of who we have been, as understood through our lived experiences, and in that process the conscious self may evolve. This process of self-evolution through self-reflection is characterized by a perception of temporal transfusion where past is merged with the present and future in one continuum.

Irene[1] was one of the cognitively intact residents I interviewed. As she was recollecting her childhood years on a Nebraska farm, she reminisced about mealtime in their home. The recollection was not only very detailed in the physical aspects of the dining space and furniture, but also as clear as if she were actually visualizing that scene now and here. She used her hands to point out in space where the dining table was and who sat where, and she described the conversations. I could sense that, for her, the remembering of that time and place was very real and immediate. The present-tense verbs in her recollection and her vivid description almost made me "see" the place with her. But all the time she was talking, she was in present time, not just physically, but also in her mind as she mentioned the comparative option of mealtimes in present days. In Irene's words:

> Oh, mealtime was the only way you could see everybody. . . . Everybody was home from school or whatever activity they attended. You didn't have fast food and stop-off joints. Oh yes, I can see this—my mother is saying—come in, come in, girls, Betty, Lucille, come in and set the table.

It's time to do that. We come in and get the dishes out and set the places for everybody. Is so and so gonna be here tonight? Yeah, he's gonna be here. And so there is a place set, and if some unexpected stranger or company got in or if somebody happened to be dropping in at that time, the preacher could come in. Then you move the plates around and put another setting on the table. The head of the family will sit there and mother will sit closest to the stove where she could replenish the dishes, the serving dishes, and each child had a different place. It is a long table of mahogany with rounded corners. Almost ten people can sit there. Yes, very definitely. Everybody will have his or her seat. And–get out of my seat, if you sat in the wrong seat.

I suggest that the functions of memory and place are strikingly parallel–both perform the same task of *threading together the disparate into a subjective unity.* A place contextualizes life experiences. Home, most often, is the physical context that holds together many diverse events that occur over time in one's life but are related to that place. It embodies in its symbolic strength all that is subjectively meaningful. In memory–or rather in the act of remembering–the diverse moments of times are drawn together. The past becomes relevant in the present, and in its contextual reality, the present becomes part of the past. In remembering, we go through a temporal transfusion, or synthesis. Within this parallelism of memory and place can we appreciate the power of remembering places. To remember particular places from our past or to remember by means of place, we can intensify our power of remembering as a journey in time. Memories of places promise temporal synthesis to the second power.

THE ENDURING "SELF"

Psychological well-being is the ultimate outcome in a causal model of the open type. It may be defined as the weighted evaluated level of the person's competence and perceived quality in all domains of contemporary life. The "weighted" aspect of this definition implies that *psychological well-being is more than a simple sum of competencies and satisfactions.* To explain the weighting process requires yet another conceptual superstructure, the self, which is a schema formed by proactive and reactive processes that provides a template for interpreting all aspects of past, present, and future experience. [italics added] (Lawton, 1991, p. 11)

Although Powell Lawton did not explicitly address the concept of "self" at great length, the significance and relevance of self as an integrating concept in understanding psychological well-being is very clear from the above para-phrase. He emphasized the importance of objective, subjective and consensual understanding in experience of the environment. Moving beyond the signifi-cance objective and discrete aspects of the environment, he pointed out the transactional nature of person-environment interaction, as well as its subjec-tive nature. In conceptualizing the place-based reminiscence process, the "self" plays the crucial integrating role. Although there are clearly identifiable social and shared dimensions of reminiscence activity, it is by and large an in-dividual process where the self is reflected upon, recollected from the past, and recreated or preserved in the present. The status of self as having both "I"–as subject–and "Me"–as object–is of suspect in a person effected by the progres-sive conditions of dementia. The social aspect of the self "Me," based upon memories of past life experiences can be considered to be fragmented, eroded, and inaccessible. The process of recollection of the personal past as an interac-tive process between these two aspects (I-Me) of self becomes disconnected and fragile.

In the progressive stages of dementia, the person moves from minor lapses in memory, to conscious effort in compensating memory loss, to cognitive and behavioral difficulties associated with loss of memory. The social self be-comes eroded by the gradual regression of memory toward early years. This aspect of the "Me" goes back in time and expresses itself, among other things, through expressions by residents with dementia in a nursing home, "I want to go home," where the home she or he refers to is that of the childhood home. Also, the inability of the self in dementia to see itself as an "object" relates to the inaccessible nature of the "Me." The internal dialogue between these "I" and "Me" of the self can be conceptualized as an ongoing reminiscence pro-cess. This process represents the inner evolution of the present "I" based on continuous validation by the past "Me." The "I" becomes "Me" and the "Me" feeds into the "I" in this process of recollection that remains, for the most part, underneath the self-consciousness.

My exploratory study on place-therapy had an initial hypothesis in this re-gard that the process of this ongoing validation of the "I" in its ability to see it-self as an object is impaired in dementia. The conditions of dementia result in a discontinuation of this "I-Me" or subject-object identification and validation. Based on the conversations with residents with dementia, it was apparent that residents' verbal and visual prompts triggered their recollections to the extent it was elicited. I suggest that the place-related information from the personal past, in verbal and visual form, provided surrogates of the "Me" that is presum-ably impaired in the self in dementia. The prompts helped the subjective aspect of self "I" to be reflexive, and identify itself as an object to itself and aid in the recollection process. Moreover, the sharing of that recollection to others offers the opportunity to reestablish the social experience that represents the original social experience which gave rise to social aspect of the self "Me" in the first place. Verbal sharing of recalled experiences could allow the individual to go beyond the "I" and reach out to the "Me" as the process of recollection evolves.

PLURALITY IN METHOD

If we conceive of person-environment relationships as being arranged in hierarchical order of complexity the specificity of a relationship confirmed at one level may not be preserved on the next. Thus the units of causal relationships at lower levels are frequently transformed into more complex units that include the lower level units but require new concepts or methods we shall argue that more complex levels require more global concepts and that, for the present, qualitative approaches to empirical research are better able to deal with such concepts. (Parmelee & Lawton, 1990, pp. 476-477)

Is there any chance that we can even measure a construct (QOL) so complex? I say we can if we respect its complexity. (Lawton, 1997, p. 45)

Evolution is a natural progression–in personal life as well as in intellectual thinking. Lawton (1982, 2000) commented on how the ecological model (Lawton & Nahemow, 1973) could be improved by recognizing the people's needs and preferences, along with their competencies. His "quality of life" model is much broader in its scope of person-environment interaction in recognition of the fact that environment is characterized not only by demands but by resources and opportunities, and behavioral competence and perceived quality of life are central in understanding quality of life. From a methodological standpoint, as noted by the above-mentioned paraphrase, Lawton was appreciative of the value of qualitative approaches in enriching our understanding of the complexity of both objective and subjective evaluation of the environment. Although, his own empirical work primarily employed quantitative methodological designs, Lawton's (Parmelee & Lawton, 1990) epistemological position is marked with recognition and support for plurality. My study on place-based reminiscence–with its potential in improving the quality of lives for residents in long-term care settings–was intellectually inspired by such a position.

Qualitative research in place attachment or place experience literature is sparse. With some few notable exceptions (e.g., Rowles, 1983; Rubinstein, 1989), there is a lack of studies looking at place experience from a more naturalistic perspective–to understand the richness, complexities, and fine-grained nuances of the phenomenon. The study on "place-based reminiscence" is based on the fundamental issue of complexity and holistic nature of human experience. The concept of "place" is considered as socially constructed, yet environmentally embedded. In order to tap into the richness of residents' past place experiences, there need to be explicit recognition of the integrality of social-personal life events within the context of physical environments. The study was built upon a qualitative research approach with a number of assumptions that informed the exploration. Although these ontological and epistemological assumptions may be somewhat *a priori* in a qualitative study, I feel that making them explicit can help the reader orient the study within this context.

First, the basic assumption in this study is that recollection of the past is a creative and dynamic process. We can consider "experience" as referring to the processes of thinking, feeling, acting aided by subjective perception, beliefs and attitudes. Human experience is broader and deeper than the "empirical" truth. Empiricism validates truth in terms of sense experience. The subjective elements–including preference, beliefs, attitudes, values, intuition and intentions–all interact in shaping the nature of our experience. In this sense, all human experience is a product of objective "reality" as well as, subjective implications. Over time, the initial experience gains new meaning and nuances. As the person evolves in life through various life stages and life experiences, recollection of past experience is filtered through his or her changing physical, psychological and social circumstances. On another level, as the recollection is shared with me, the residents' lived experience was also filtered through my individual perception and understanding and once again gained an added layer of interpretation.

A second assumption underlying the study's methodology is that in the experience of places, the self is associated with the place in a "transactional" manner. This "transactional" world view (Altman & Rogoff, 1987; Pepper, 1967; Dewey & Bentley, 1949) has the following essential features: (a) people and psychological processes are embedded in and inseparable from their physical and social contexts; (b) temporal qualities are inherent aspects of phenomena; (c) there are multiple levels of realities. To understand the self in place, one would look at the interaction and experience of the place with other events and individuals. Place as part of individual experience and recollection is influenced and mediated by other individuals and social processes.

The final assumption is that in a qualitative inquiry such as this, a reality (one of many realities) is created as opposed to being discovered. There is no single reality out there to be discovered by the researcher. Meaning is created through interpretative processes that involve looking at the phenomenon under study with *positionality* and *structural embeddedness* (Jaffe & Miller, 1994).

"Positionality" refers to identity and worldview of the researcher, the subjects of the research, and "structural embeddedness" refers to the relationship between the phenomenon and the broader social context. The process of making meaning is influenced by the dynamic interplay of positionality and structural embeddedness. For example, an individual "positionality" that views the experience of aging with fear may find it difficult to accept the "structural embeddedness" approach that advocates age-integrated residential environments.

SUBJECTIVE NATURE OF QUALITY OF LIFE

The *intrapersonal* aspects of quality of life express one essential ingredient of a comprehensive conception, that each individual has internal standards and evaluations of life that are idiosyncratic and not totally accountable to any external standard. Many conceptions of quality of life depend solely upon subjective evaluations for the definition of quality. (Lawton, 1991, p. 7)

Subjective perception of quality of life is a central dimension in Powell Lawton's (1991) quality of life model. He insisted on consideration of both objective and subjective evaluations of the environment. If psychological well-being is the aspired outcome of caring for the elderly in long-term care settings, it is crucial that we take into account the residents' personal preferences, attitudes and feelings, toward understanding and supporting the self-identity. Throughout life, the past helps us maintain a coherent sense of self amidst the physical, social and psychological changes that come with old age, dementia and relocation to an institution.

In recollection of the past, the temporal boundaries of the past and present get blurred (Chaudhury, 1999; Tobin, 1991). Personally meaningful past place experiences, in the process of recall, is a transforming process that makes one relive the past with all its sensory experiences, social context and affective connotations. This is a dynamic process of subjective recreation of the past that does not duplicate the historical truth, but rather reflects a process that has been primarily meaningful at the individual level. It is a reflection of human desire and the innate need for finding meaning or creating meaning in the world around us. In this meaning-making process, places provide structure and anchors for the stream of lived experiences. We cannot live without meaning, and creating meaning through places is a natural process of being human without which life would largely remain two-dimensional. And as place experience becomes an integral part of one's internal landscape, the outer becomes inner.

This is a landscape of perception, preference, deep attachment, joy, love, longing, fear, and sense of loss.

On the other hand, the "substance" of our inner lives gets reflected in our outer environment. The unfamiliar places gradually become part of ourselves as we expand our inner energy outward. For example, the experience of moving to a new city is disorienting, and places are strange in the beginning–devoid of one's own experience. But over time, we become familiar with places, we create rituals, we inhabit and in this process–carved into the mosaic of time–places take on an inner dimension. In this dynamic process our experiential world expands, and we become more at home in a larger environment. The landscape around us is created, to a greater or lesser extent, by the way in which we are defined to ourselves and by others.

I suggest that in this process of outer and inner landscapes being intertwined, the place and self become one. The reality of the physical boundaries of an individual and place dissolves in the transference of self to the place and the place to the self. The physical dichotomy gives way to an imaginative integration. In remembering the past, we remember the events, people, and places–all part of the same image. As Poulet (1977) comments:

> Beings surround themselves with the places where they find themselves, the way one wraps oneself up in a garment that is at one and the same time a disguise and characterization. Without places, beings would be abstractions. It is places that make their image precise and that give them the necessary support thanks to which we can assign them a place in our mental place, dream of them and remember them. (p. 26)

This phenomenon of deep interpenetration of places and selves is far too deep to be captured in an excerpt. However, this aspect does surface in people's reflections on place–as it has in some reflective reminiscing among the residents I interviewed. For instance, Irene remembered her childhood homes and she talked about the trees in the backyard. As she visualized the trees, she became reflective and expressed her deep association with one of the trees. Without going into analysis of the premise or context of her self-association with a tree, one can appreciate this as an illustration of her imagination through which childhood feelings were transfused with those of a tree. As one of the residents Irene reflected:

> I think the house I grew up in on the north side, the house was a little away from the street and we had apple trees on the backyard. I remember there was one tree that was smaller than the others and I used to think that was me. I liked the trees very much and specially that smaller one. It

grew under the shade of a big tree–maybe that's why it was small. I could almost feel how that tree was feeling.

On the other hand, another resident (Kate's) reflection on the services held in her nursing home points out how the outer landscape can remind her of her own values and philosophy. Kate did not appreciate the services of the nursing home, not because she was not religious, but rather because the way they were conducted was something she was not used to. The activity and, consequently, the place didn't reflect her and she chose not to be part of that. In Kate's words:

> I shouldn't say it, but this is quite Orthodox. I'm not used to that. See here . . . the men and women are separated. The men, they sit in front, and the women sit in back. I don't go, I'm sorry. I'm not used to that. This is quite an Orthodox place. I shouldn't say. But I don't like the segregation. This place is not me. I was brought up, well my parents were Orthodox, but not that strict as here.

Whether a place resonates in one's self or not is a matter of specific individual and place contexts. However, the process of discovery is primarily the same; we seek out reflections of our preferences, values, and beliefs in the places where we are. I suggest that place-oriented recollection represents a journey concerning place, self and remembering, how they relate to each other and as a holistic experiential phenomenon. In general terms, the idea of *journey* brings up notions of travel (whether seriously undertaken migrations, or mere pleasure trips) through geographic landscape–going from one place to another. The term *journey* encompasses this basic conception of physical movement, as well as two others aspects. These latter aspects of journey relate to time and self. The activity of remembering past places and associated life experiences refer to the primacy of time. Respondents in the study journeyed back into time to retrieve memories of places, events and people. Although the physical self remained in present time, remembering the past was a conscious effort of moving away from the present time and focusing attention on a different time. Also, journey reflects a journey of the self in its reflexivity to see itself as an object. In remembering the past, the "I" of self identified itself in the past as an "object." In this identification and association, the "I" reaffirms itself to itself in an evolving journey. Mindful remembering of one's own past is a process that reminds oneself of what who one was then, and how that relates to how one is now.

I suggest that all three dimensions of the journey also reflect a self-evolution in the sense in each act of recall there are two sets of "places," "times," and "selves." Recollecting a place from one's past brings to surface a place that is not identical, but *identifiable* to what the person actually experienced in the original time. The childhood home that is *recollected* is not in its entirety, but signifies its fragmented and highlighted portions that the person remembers. Memories of the home bring up descriptions of physical features and social contexts that are not photographic images of the historical home, but are personal reconstruction of the place. At a temporal level, recollections are about the *past* that occurs in the *present*. Likewise, the *self* carrying out the recollection is not the identical *self* of the past. The elderly resident who recollected her childhood home is no longer the child who had the original experience of the home. The passage of time aside, it is the accumulated life experiences that have influenced the child-self into becoming her late-adult-self.

WHAT LIES AHEAD?

Although Lawton's quality of life conceptual model was not explicitly adopted in the place-based reminiscence study, it was the guiding track. The study provides support that personally meaningful places can be used in remembering life experiences and which in turn, can provide a sense of continuity for residents in nursing homes. The process has potential in affirmation of self-identity and achieving congruence between expected and achieved goals in life among cognitively intact older adults, and in turn, can improve their quality of life. The efficacy of place-oriented recollection for positive outcomes in the quality of life for residents need to be further explored. A particular challenge with place-therapy lies in working with people with dementia in preservation of their sense of selves. This is a goal that directly relates to the desired "good life" that Lawton espoused. I would propose three avenues toward further exploration in the efficacy of place-therapy for older adults in long-term care settings. These are conceptually and substantively overlapping with the singular goal of enhancing the quality of life of residents through recognition, affirmation, and preservation of the self.

- *Recognize the unique subjectivity of residents:* This is at the core of place-therapy approach. The dominant paradigm for caring for physically and cognitively impaired institutionalized elderly is couched in the medical model that defines and shapes personal identity and worth through physiological conditions. Place-therapy begins with the fundamental premise that each person is unique with her or his own personal life stories that must be gathered, appreciated and affirmed.
- *"Remembering" as repository for experiences, rather than repository of experiences:* Recollection of the past through personally experienced

places advocate celebrating the past not in a nostalgic mode of remembering. Rather the prime objective is putting past to work in the present. The very process of remembering and sharing is viewed as a source of new experience. This is a dynamic process that involves recruitment of memories, thoughts, actions and feelings within the current perceptions where early events affect current perceptions, and in turn, current perceptions may affect the reconstruction of the past.

* *Involving family members in developing place-biosketches, activity planning and practice:* Biographical knowledge of residents with dementia can be incorporated into care planning and practice (Chaudhury, in press). Especially for residents with dementia, as the sense of identity gradually becomes inaccessible, place-biosketches could be a tool in holding on to the sense of self. Family members of residents with dementia can be involved in developing place-biosketches, as well as in planning and conducting activities based on the collected information that are personally meaningful to the residents.

Much needs to be explored in assessing the efficacy of place-therapy on potential affective and/or cognitive impact. As with any other therapeutic activity, place-therapy sessions need to be an ongoing activity for evaluation of the intervention. Group versus one-on-one sessions, as well as the cognitive status of residents would likely have variable efficacy in eliciting recollection. In this essay I have attempted to propose place-therapy as a potential therapeutic activity within the conceptual framework of quality of life. The fundamental recognition of the self at the core of four sectors in QOL model provides the support for understanding the self in old age and in dementia, and for developing ways in which we can respect the complexity of the concept of QOL in older individuals.

NOTE

1. All names of residents and places are pseudonyms.

REFERENCES

Altman, I. & Rogoff, B. (1987). World views in psychology: Trait, interactional, organismic, and transactional perspectives. In D. Stokols & I. Altman (Eds.), *Handbook of environmental psychology* (pp. 7-40). New York: Wiley.

Chaudhury, H. (1999). Self and Reminiscence of Place: A Conceptual Study. *The Journal of Aging & Identity, 4*(4), 231-254.

Chaudhury, H. (in press). Journey back home: Recollecting past places by people with dementia. *Journal of Housing for the Elderly.*

Chaudhury, H. (in press). Place-biosketch as a tool in caring for people with dementia. *Alzheimer's Care Quarterly.*

Dewey, J. & Bentley, A. F. (1949). *Knowing and the known.* Boston, MA: Beacon.

Gibson, F. (1994). What can reminiscence contribute to people with dementia. In J. Bornat (Ed.), *Reminiscence reviewed: Evaluations, achievements, perspectives* (pp. 46-60). Buckingham: Open University Press.

Jaffe, D. J. & Miller, E. M. (1994). Problematizing meaning. In J. F. Gubrium and A. Sankar (Eds.), *Qualitative methods in aging research* (pp. 51-64). Thousand Oaks, CA: Sage Publications.

James, W. (1892). *Psychology: The briefer course.* New York: Henry Holt.

Kitwood, T. (1997). *Dementia reconsidered: The person comes first.* Buckingham: Open University Press.

Lawton, M. P. (1982). Competence, environmental press, and the adaptation of older people. In M. P. Lawton, P. G. Windley, & T. O. Byerts (Eds.), *Aging and the environment: Theoretical approaches* (pp. 33-59). New York: Springer.

Lawton, M.P. (1991). A multidimensional view of quality of life in frail elders. In J. E. Birren, J. E. Lubben, J. C. Rowe, & D. E. Deutchman (Eds.), *The concept and measurement of quality of life in the frail elderly* (pp. 3-27). New York: Academic Press.

Lawton, M.P. (1997). Measures of quality of life and subjective well-being. *Generations,* 21(1), 45-47.

Lawton, M.P. (2000). Chance and choice make a good life. In. J. E. Birren and J. F. Schroots (Eds.), *A history of geropsychology in autobiography* (pp. 185-196). Washington, DC: American Psychological Association.

Lawton, M. P. & Nahemow, L. (1973). Ecology and the aging process. In C. Eisdorfer & M. P. Lawton (Eds.), *Psychology of adult development and aging* (pp. 619-624). Washington, DC: American Psychological Association.

Mead, G. H. (1934). *Mind, self and society.* Chicago: University of Chicago Press.

Parmelee, P. A. & Lawton, M. P. (1990). The design of special environments for the aged. In J. E. Birren & K. W. Schaie (Eds.), *Handbook of the Psychology of Aging* (pp. 464-488). San Diego, CA: Academic Press.

Pepper, S. C. (1967). *World hypotheses.* Berkeley, CA: University of California Press.

Piper, A. I. & Langer, E. J. (1986). Aging and mindful control. In M. M. Baltes & P. B. Baltes (Eds.), *The psychology of control and aging* (pp. 71-89). Hillsdale, NJ: Erlbaum.

Poulet, G. (1977). *Proustian space.* Baltimore: Johns Hopkins University Press.

Rosenmayr, L. (1982). Biography and identity. In T. K. Harevan and K. J. Adams (Eds.), *Aging and life course transitions: An interdisciplinary perspective* (pp. 27-53). New York: Guilford Press.

Rowles, G. D. (1983). Place and personal identity in old age: Observations from Appalachia. *Journal of Environmental Psychology,* 3, 299-313.

Rubinstein, R. L. (1989). The home environments of older people: A description of psychological processes linking person to place. *Journal of Gerontology,* 44, S45-S53.

Rubinstein, R. L. & Parmelee, P. A. (1992). Attachment to place and the representation of the life course by the elderly. In I. Altman & S. M. Low (Eds.), *Place attachment* (pp. 139-163). New York: Plenum.

Tobin, S. S. (1991). *Personhood in advanced old age: Implications for practice.* New York: Springer.

Weisman, G.D., Chaudhury, H., & Moore, K.D. (2000). Theory and Practice of Place: Toward an Integrative Model. In R. Rubinstein, M. Moss, & M. Kleban (Eds.), *The many dimensions of aging: Essays in honor of M. Powell Lawton* (pp. 3-21). Springer.

Woods, B. & McKiernan (1995). Evaluating the impact of reminiscence on older people with dementia. In B. K. Haight & J. D. Webster (Eds.), *The art and science of reminiscing: Theory, research, methods, and applications.* (pp. 233-242). Washington, DC: Taylor & Francis.

Advancements
in the Home Modification Field:
A Tribute to M. Powell Lawton

Jon Pynoos
Christy Nishita
Lena Perelman

SUMMARY. M. Powell Lawton can be credited for important advancements in the home modification field. His work extended beyond theoretical contributions to practical efforts that directly impact older adults' lives. Developments in home modification research, assessment approaches, and the service delivery system can be attributed to his influence. Lawton's efforts shaped the home modification field with the recognition that a supportive physical environment can enable an older adult to successfully adapt to declining functional abilities. *[Article copies available for a fee from The Haworth Document Delivery Service: 1-800-HAWORTH. E-mail address: <getinfo@haworthpressinc.com> Website: <http://www.HaworthPress.com> © 2003 by The Haworth Press, Inc. All rights reserved.]*

KEYWORDS. Home modification, aging-in-place, competence-press

INTRODUCTION

M. Powell Lawton's contributions over his lifetime have been far-reaching and influential. His work in theory development has had a tremendous impact

---

Jon Pynoos, Christy Nishita, and Lena Perelman are affiliated with the University of Southern California.

[Haworth co-indexing entry note]: "Advancements in the Home Modification Field: A Tribute to M. Powell Lawton." Pynoos, Jon, Nishita, Christy, and Perelman, Lena. Co-published simultaneously in *Journal of Housing for the Elderly* (The Haworth Press, Inc.) Vol. 17, No. 1/2, 2003, pp. 105-116; and: *Physical Environments and Aging: Critical Contributions of M. Powell Lawton to Theory and Practice* (ed: Rick J. Scheidt, and Paul G. Windley) The Haworth Press, Inc., 2003, pp. 105-116. Single or multiple copies of this article are available for a fee from The Haworth Document Delivery Service [1-800-HAWORTH, 9:00 a.m. - 5:00 p.m. (EST). E-mail address: getinfo@haworthpressinc.com].

on the field. But his focus moved beyond theoretical concerns to an effort to directly improve the lives of older adults. Lawton recognized that the majority of elderly lived independently in their own homes and preferred to continue this way for as long as possible. He applied his abstract conceptualizations to practical concerns of design, assessment, and the development of best practices to facilitate "aging in place." His focus on the physical environment fostered the growth of the home modification field, which recognizes the impact of modifying or adapting the home on maintaining independence. While Lawton's contributions are vast, this article focuses on his influence on the home modifications field and its service delivery system.

IMPACT ON THE HOME MODIFICATION FIELD

Instead of facilitating older persons' ability to grow old safely, independently, and with dignity, many homes have instead become a source of the problem itself. Maintaining control, independence, and privacy are primary concerns of older adults. Lawton brought attention to the importance of the physical environment in facilitating "aging in place." He addressed the need for housing to be "usable" (Lawton, 1985) and "accommodating."

The key to aging in place is maintaining the right fit between a person's abilities and the demands of the environment. Lawton and Nahemow's (1973) competence-press model asserts that adaptive behavior involves the balance between one's internal abilities (competence) and forces in the environment that place demands on an individual (press). A number of researchers have attempted to operationalize the competence-press model. For example, Pynoos and Regnier (1991) developed 12 environment-behavior principles, such as privacy, social interaction, autonomy, aesthetics, orientation, safety, and adaptability. These principles can be used to create a research framework that is sensitive to the range and types of decisions made by designers and policymakers. They represent a means through which social science-based research can more tangibly influence management, program, policy, and design areas.

A mismatch between functional ability and the environment can lead to excess disability. For example, an older person who has problems with mobility and lower body strength may not be able to climb the flight of stairs in his/her home. Similarly, a person who has trouble with flexibility, reaching, or grasping may have difficulty using conventional round door knobs.

Reducing excess disability involves either improving the abilities of the person or reducing the demand of the environment. Too often, older persons adapt their behaviors to their environments rather than change their settings to meet their needs. Even professionals such as doctors, occupational therapists, or case managers overlook the role of the environment in supporting frail older persons (Verbrugge & Jette, 1993). There is a growing consensus that interventions such as home modifications may prevent, minimize, or reverse disablement outcomes (Verbrugge & Jette, 1993).

Home modifications are environmental adaptations aimed at creating a more supportive environment, enhancing participation in major life activities, preventing accidents, facilitating caregiving, and minimizing the need for more costly personal care services (Pynoos, Tabbarah, Angelelli, & Demiere, 1998). There are five ways older persons can adapt to the environment or change the environment itself to meet their needs: structural changes, special equipment, assistive devices, material adjustments, and behavioral changes (Pynoos, Cohen, Davis, & Bernhardt, 1987). Modifications to existing environments can range and vary from structural changes such as door widening and installation of ramps to specialized equipment that includes grab bars, handrails, and shower benches.

Assessing the Magnitude of the Problem

Lawton was concerned with assessing the nature and magnitude of older adults' housing needs. His publications utilized statistics to highlight current status and unmet need (Lawton, 1985). Yet, he pointed out a crucial flaw in national datasets. Datasets, such as the American Housing Survey, considered a dwelling unit of good quality if it did not have any deficiencies or need for repair. However, front steps in good condition are insufficient if the person has ambulatory problems and still cannot get in and out of the house. Lawton asserted that true housing quality involved consideration of the user's needs and abilities (Lawton, 1985).

Up until recently, national datasets did not recognize that persons were modifying homes to accommodate their functional limitations. Gradually, supplements to the American Housing Survey have measured the presence of home modification features such as handrails, grab bars, ramps, easy access bathrooms, and easy access kitchens. In addition, national datasets such as the National Long-Term Care Survey and the Survey of Asset and Health Dynamics have included items related to home modification, allowing researchers to examine its prevalence, remaining unmet need, and effectiveness.

Research indicates a rising prevalence in the use of home modifications. Between 1982-1989 the National Long-Term Care Survey of community-dwelling older persons ages 65 or over has documented large increases in the use of assistive devices and home modifications. The most rapidly increasing items included raised toilet seats (148%), shower seat/tub stools (65.9%), grab bars (64.9%) and portable toilets (30.7%) (Manton, Corder, & Stallard, 1993). The increase in use of assistive devices and home modifications was accompanied by a decline in the use of personal assistance by older respondents with physical impairments. The results suggest that home modifications substitute for personal care services, but the mechanism is unclear. Estimates of the National Center for Health Care Statistics indicate that 7.1 million persons live in homes that have special features for those with impairments (LaPlante, Hendershot, & Moss, 1992). In conventional homes and apartments, grab bars and shower seats were the most common home modification reported by almost a quarter of the population (22.9%), followed by wheelchair accessibility within the home (9.0%), railings (7.8%), and ramps at street level (5.0%) (Tabarrah, Silverstein, & Seeman, 2000).

Lawton's influence also contributed to consumer studies focused exclusively on home modifications. AARP consulted Lawton about questions to include in developing a survey on housing and home modification issues (AARP, 2000). Findings from the study indicate that many Americans over age 45 use home modifications to make their home easier to live in. The most prevalent modifications include installing light switches in stairwells to reduce the likelihood of falls and making modifications to enable persons to live on the first floor. Simple changes are also made such as nightlights and non-skid bathtub strips. The majority of persons who made modifications felt that these changes would enable them to remain at home longer.

Nevertheless, research suggests that an unmet need exists among individuals who would benefit from environmental modifications. Of the existing 100 million residential units, fewer than 10 percent have home modification features in them (LaPlante et al., 1992). Over five million older households have one household member with a functional limitation. According to HUD data, of these, almost half (2.1 million) express the need for home modifications to function independently, while only 1.14 million of these households have the modifications they desire (Joint Center for Housing Studies, 2000). If current demographic and population trends continue, the existing gap between individuals who would benefit from accessible housing and the available accessible housing units will multiply (Pynoos et al., 1998).

IMPACT OF HOME MODIFICATIONS ON SERVICE DELIVERY

Lawton recognized that the delivery of home modification services is important given that the majority of older adults live independently (Lawton, 1985). Yet, the increasing need of frail older adults and younger persons with disabilities for home modifications has not yet been matched by an adequate service delivery system. The most frequently cited reasons for not making home modifications are that older adults are unable to do it themselves, they cannot afford it, and they do not trust home contractors (AARP, 2000).

Two decades ago, Lawton described the service delivery system as a "patchwork" of public and private programs and providers, funding from federal, state, local, and private sources, and the various governmental agencies involved in administering funds (Lawton, 1985; Saperstein et al., 1986). The service delivery system still suffers from many of the same problems. It can be characterized as a mixed array of services involving a variety of groups and individuals, range and types of home modifications, and approaches to service delivery (Pynoos et al., 1998).

Assessment Needs

An important first step in the home modification process is a proper assessment of the home. The process involves identifying the person's functional limitations that make performing daily tasks difficult, barriers in the environment, and the interaction between the two (Pynoos, Sanford, & Rosenfeld, in press). Yet the process is not standardized in that many assessors are not adequately trained and most assessment instruments are simple checklists. Some building professionals perform assessments without the benefit of a formal instrument. Even occupational therapists may employ inadequate assessment instruments and have difficulties integrating home modifications into their care plans.

In the mid-1980s, Lawton recognized a lack of housing expertise among social service workers. He considered it unlikely that large scale, national home modification programs would be created. Instead, he aimed to improve the housing expertise of existing social service agencies. Along with colleagues at the Philadelphia Geriatric Center, he developed a specific assessment instrument to enhance the skills of professionals to assess the qualities of the client's home (Saperstein et al., 1986).

THE ROLE OF HOME MODIFICATION PROGRAMS

Given the difficulties in securing an accurate assessment and other services, home modification programs have developed to provide the range of providers and services needed to complete the home modification process. Hundreds of home modification programs are in existence across the country (National Resource and Policy Center, 1998), representing two basic types of service delivery: non-profit and for-profit. In the past two decades, the number of non-profit programs has increased along with for-profit home modification companies. Both for-profit companies and non-profit organizations have generally the same mission: to assist older adults and persons with disabilities remain independent. Nevertheless, they are different in several ways.

Non-profit agencies target those most in need, including ethnic minorities and low-income elderly. Their assessments focus on the functional abilities of clients as well as the environment and are usually conducted by individuals with a construction or occupational therapy/physical therapy background. In comparison, the for-profit companies are geared towards persons who can pay. Assessment usually focuses on the structural elements of the home environment and is in direct response to the requests of the consumer. Thus, for-profit companies respond mainly to the particular problems of the client rather than comprehensively examining the fit between person and environment. Whether this approach is disadvantageous to the client is unclear.

The differing funding/revenue sources produce strong distinctions between the two types of models. Inadequate funding for non-profit organizations limits the number and types of home modifications they can provide. They can often only perform small jobs in order to maximize the number of persons they can serve. Unlike non-profit counterparts, for-profit companies often have the capabilities to implement major modifications upon the request of its clients. Because for-profit companies obtain much of its revenue from large modification jobs, they are often reluctant to accept small jobs due to their low profitability.

Problems with Current Home Modification Programs

Despite the availability of two types of service delivery, there are significant geographical gaps in services and many programs suffer from long waiting lists. Programs vary in the kinds and range of services they provide, their methods of assessment, and funding (Pynoos et al., 1998). Many programs provide mainly home maintenance and repair, and only recently have added home modifications in response to a newly recognized need.

Programs providing home modifications have difficulty securing and maintaining adequate funding. Often, they must piece together funding from different sources, such as government funds, private foundations, fundraising, and individual donations. Some programs such as Rebuild America and Habitat for Humanity rely extensively on volunteers. Programs often find that demand for services outweighs their available funding, especially in relation to providing more costly modifications such as stair glides, walk-in showers, and bathroom redesign.

Without dedication to the provision of home modifications and a lack of stability in funding for home modification, many programs do not have sufficient expertise in this area. They may not have the proper tools or knowledge to accurately assess both the needs of the person as well as the environment. Many programs are small in scale and lack the resources to expand their presence in the community. Joint funding and projects with other agencies and alliances with disability, housing, and health care groups can promote knowledge and awareness within the community.

One approach to addressing these problems is to identify best practices in home modification programs that can serve as models. Lawton's work demonstrated a deep interest in describing best practices in planning and developing senior housing. He emphasized locating housing in safe neighborhoods with proximity to parks, transportation, and services. Using photographs and architectural plans, optimal approaches to designing safe, functional, and accessible housing units were identified. Lawton emphasized that these factors would lead to "successful adjustment," by enabling older adults to operate within their physical environment (Lawton, 1975). The following section extends Lawton's efforts by identifying best practices in home modification programs.

Best Practices in Home Modification Programs

Lawton laid the groundwork for innovation in the home modification field by identifying problems and suggesting approaches to address these problems. Lawton recognized that older adults require suitable and appropriate housing. Such housing went beyond bricks and mortar to a setting that accommodated declining functional ability. He viewed home modifications as an approach to reducing the demand of one's physical environment. He regarded data sets as inadequate, leading to the revision of national data sets and the increase of home modification research. Such research has demonstrated how important the environment may be for older persons. However, serving this population requires the availability of adequate assessments and a coordinated service delivery system. Recognizing that a national program is unlikely, he focused on strengthening existing social service agencies by improving their supportive housing expertise. In summary, Lawton's contribution to the field was his identification of the importance of system integration, research, and appropriate assessments. Home modification programs have developed exemplary approaches in these areas.

System Integration

System integration is an innovative approach to address the patchwork service delivery system problem identified by Lawton. For example, the South

East Senior Housing Initiative (SESHI) is a coalition of various organizations within the South East Baltimore community. Together, these collaborators work to promote independent living among the senior population by creating a network of referral agencies and providers. The members recognize the importance of sharing information and contributing services to keep seniors in their community safe and healthy. The coalition, from its inception, has utilized community organizations, citizens, and resources to contribute to the network of services, program design, and implementation.

Inter-agency partnerships are created under the SESHI coalition. These agencies make referrals to each other to bring together many services already available but which many seniors access in a haphazard or discontinuous manner. While SESHI refers to a coalition, there is a SESHI office with a small staff that organizes the coalition's activities. The SESHI office acts like a case manager, providing clients with the appropriate information and services. For instance, a client may contact SESHI because they need environmental adaptations to make it easier to take a bath. SESHI will then set up an appointment with an OT to conduct an in-home assessment and refer the client to an agency that can implement the needed modifications.

The Philadelphia Corporation on Aging (PCA) in Philadelphia, PA represents a model of intra-agency coordination. Social workers, the first point of contact for clients of the home modification program, look not only at the home but at other client needs as well. They often make referrals to other programs within PCA such as Meals-on-Wheels, or other programs in the community. They are able to pull together four to five funding sources such as Pennsylvania General Funds and Community Development Block Grants to address as many of the client's needs as possible. Within the Housing Department of PCA, a team approach involves the cooperation of the consumer, OT, and builder to maximize the functioning of the consumer within their home environment. In such a collaboration, each partner contributes his/her knowledge and skills throughout the home modification delivery process.

RESEARCHING THE EFFECTIVENESS
OF HOME MODIFICATIONS

Another innovative development is that some programs are conducting research to test the effectiveness of home modifications. PCA administers two home modification programs that served 750 homes in the last year. PCA provides researchers at Thomas Jefferson University with access to its clients and installs home modifications for clinical intervention studies that examine the effectiveness of home modifications.

SESHI is in the process of implementing a new Robert Woods Johnson Foundation grant that will last four years. The research component of the grant will attempt to assess the extent to which providing home modifications prior to injury is a cost effective means that prevents nursing home placement. SESHI hopes that positive results will help convince the medical community and insurance groups of the importance of home modifications.

Assessment Protocols

Assessment is an important part of the service delivery process. Accurate assessments are needed to ensure that the modifications fit the specific needs and capabilities of the individual. Lawton was an early pioneer in assessing the environment, health, and functional ability (Saperstein et al., 1986; Kovar & Lawton, 1994). He advocated a continued exploration of new methodologies to determine the most appropriate method for asking questions and reducing measurement error (Kovar & Lawton, 1994). He developed a framework for understanding the older person's interrelationship with his/her environment. Within this framework, he and others at the Philadelphia Geriatric Center developed a detailed room-by-room assessment checklist for the home (Saperstein et al., 1986). Lawton's concepts and process are reflected in PCA's approach to environmental assessment used in its home modification programs.

Occupational therapists (OTs) play a crucial role in the service delivery process at PCA. PCA hires OTs as consultants to assist consumers in deciding the most useful and appropriate modifications. When meeting with the client, the OT encourages the consumer to discuss his/her daily routine and identify any difficulties. By involving the older adult and his/her family in the process, they become empowered, preventing the OT from recommending items that will never be used.

Guided by a detailed checklist, the OT begins by analyzing the person and environment to gain more understanding of whom will be using the modification and for whom the modification may be a hindrance. Medical information is also collected that helps the therapists determine possible future needs or declines in functioning. Next, functional deficits are observed, as the therapist walks through the home with the client and asks he/she to simulate tasks in each area of the home. Observing the actual performance of a task is crucial because clients may not report problems in this area as they have adapted their behavior to perform the task. Moreover, most are unaware of the home modification possibilities that can benefit varying levels of functional ability.

One technique the OT employs is to distinguish between "good days" and "bad days." When asked if there is a problem performing a certain task, the client tends to respond optimistically by saying that they can do it "okay." However, when the therapist raises the possibility of a "bad day," the person may realize that the modification is needed. The intervention is designed to accommodate fluctuations in the consumer's needs without labeling the individual as incompetent. Ultimately, the OT strives to connect, understand, and meet the consumers' goals. PCA's approach has been seen as a best practice and their assessment protocol has spread to the Howard County, Maryland home modification program.

While OTs at PCA are skilled at assessing home modification needs, many others have inadequate assessment instruments or have difficulties employing home modifications in their care plans. One for-profit company has developed an assessment instrument and training guide that can assist OTs and other service providers across the country in conducting home assessments. The assessment tool fills a gap in the service delivery system by giving individuals access to assessments and solutions despite a lack of skilled providers in their own community.

Extended Home Living Services (EHLS) was established in 1991 as a private for-profit business delivering HM to younger persons with disabilities and older adults living in the Chicago suburbs. With a Small Business Innovative Research grant from the National Institute of Health, EHLS developed an assessment instrument called the Comprehensive Assessment Survey Process for Aging Residents (CASPAR) that enables service professionals to conduct accurate functional and environmental assessments. The assessment enables EHLS and other home modification specialists to provide individualized, detailed solutions without traveling to an individual's home. As a result, CASPAR can be used anywhere in the country for assessing homes and specifying modifications. It is especially useful in areas that lack trained home modification providers, but where local builders are available to construct or install the modifications recommended by EHLS or another home modification specialist.

CASPAR collects information about the client's abilities, problems, and the home environment. A service professional, such as an OT or case manager, can fill out the instrument and forward it to a home modification specialist such as EHLS. They are aided in the process by a video and an accompanying training guide. At EHLS, a staff consisting of architects, OTs, allied health professionals, and remodeling experts review the materials and consult with the client and/or service professional to develop a solution. The proposed solutions are then mailed or faxed back to the client. CASPAR, therefore, overcomes the limitations of other home assessment instruments by closing the loop among consumers, builders, and service professionals (Pynoos et al., in press).

Research finds that the use of OTs is important in the home modification process. If they are involved in the assessment process and in conducting follow-up to ensure that the work was done properly and to provide any needed training, the intervention is successful. The combination of OT's expertise and the provision of home modifications improve an older adult ability to perform daily tasks (Gitlin, Miller, & Boyce, 1999; Gitlin, Corcoran, Winter, Boyce, & Hauck, 2001).

CONCLUSION

Lawton recognized that suitable housing for the elderly extends beyond homes that are free of repair needs. The home needs to be accessible and enable older adults to perform daily life activities. His influence led to the inclusion of items in national datasets that examined not only repair needs, but also modification needs. Lawton also called attention to problems in the service delivery system. Despite continuing problems, home modification programs are developing innovative approaches to system integration, assessment, and outcomes research.

Too often, older persons adapt their behaviors to their environments rather than change their settings to meet their needs. Lawton's career demonstrates that the role of the environment should not be overlooked in its ability to support frail older persons. Home modifications can be seen as an approach that reduces the demand of the environment to create person-environment fit. Lawton has demonstrably impacted the development of the home modification field with the recognition that the physical design of the environment can encourage successful adaptation to declining functional abilities with age.

REFERENCES

AARP (2000). *Fixing to stay: A national survey of housing and home modification issues.* Washington, D.C.: AARP.

Gitlin, L.N., Corcoran, M., Winter, L., Boyce, A., & Hauck, W.W. (2001). A randomized, controlled trial of a home environmental intervention: Effect on efficacy and upset in caregivers and on daily function of persons with dementia. *Gerontologist,* 41(1), 4-14.

Gitlin, L.N., Miller, K.S., & Boyce, A. (1999). Bathroom modifications for frail elderly renters: Outcomes of a community-based program. *Technology and Disability, 10,* 141-149.

Joint Center for Housing Studies (2000). *The state of the nation's housing: 1999.* Cambridge, MA: Harvard University.

Kovar, M.G. & Lawton, M.P. (1994). Functional disability: Activities and instrumental activities of daily living. In M.P. Lawton and J.A. Teresi (Eds.). *Focus on assessment techniques: Annual review of gerontology and geriatrics* (pp. 57-75). New York: Springer Publishing Company.

La Plante, M.P., Hendershot, G.E., & Moss, A.J. (1992). Assistive technology devices and home accessibility features: Prevalence, payment, need and trends. *Advance Data*, 217, 1-12.

Lawton, M.P. (1985). Overview: Environment and its relationship to well-being. *Pride Journal of Long Term Home Health Care*, 4(2), 5-11.

Lawton, M. P. (1975). *Planning and managing housing for the elderly*. New York: John Wiley & Sons.

Lawton, M.P. & Nahemow, L. (1973). Ecology and the aging process. In C. Eisdorfer and M. P. Lawton (Eds.), *The psychology of adult development and aging* (pp. 619-674). Washington, D.C.: American Psychological Association.

Manton, K.G., Corder, L., & Stallard, E. (1993). Changes in the use of personal assistance and special equipment from 1982 to 1989: Results from the 1982 and 1989 NLTCS. *The Gerontologist*, 33(2), 168-176.

National Resource and Policy Center on Housing and Long-Term Care (1998). *National directory of home modification and repair programs*. Los Angeles: National Resource and Policy Center on Housing and Long-term Care.

Pynoos, J., Cohen, E., Davis, L., & Bernhardt, S. (1987). Home modifications: Improvements that extend independence. In V. Regnier & J. Pynoos (Eds). *Housing the aged: Design directives and policy considerations* (pp. 277-303). New York: Elsevier Science Publishing Co.

Pynoos, J. & Regnier, V. (1991). Improving residential environments for frail elderly: Bridging the gap between theory and application. In J.E. Birren, J.E. Lubben, J.C. Rowe, and D.E. Deutchman (Eds.), *The concept and measurement of quality of life in the frail elderly* (pp. 91-117). San Diego: Academic Press, Inc.

Pynoos, J. & Sanford, J., & Rosenfeld, T. (in press). Improving the delivery of home modifications to older persons. *OT Practice*.

Pynoos, J., Tabbarah, M., Angelelli, J., & Demiere, M. (1998). Improving the delivery of home modifications. *Technology and Disability*, 8, 3-14.

Saperstein, A., Lawton, M.P., Cherkas, L., Lefkowitz, C., Moleski, W.H., & Sharp, A. (1986). *A housing quality component for in-home services*. Philadelphia: Philadelphia Geriatric Center.

Tabbarah, M., Silverstein, M., & Seeman, T. (2000). A health and demographic profile of non-institutionalized older Americans residing in environments with home modifications. *Journal of Aging and Health*, 12(2), 204-228.

Verbrugge, L.M. & Jette, A.M. (1993). The disablement process. *Social Science Medicine*, 38(1), 1-14.

The Human Factors of Aging
and the Micro-Environment:
Personal Surroundings, Technology
and Product Development

Joseph A. Koncelik

SUMMARY. This article discusses how the body of knowledge designers call human factors must integrate aging as a construct for the development of environments and products. M. Powell Lawton, who
developed a significant body of knowledge about the relationship of behavior to environment, provides insight regarding this integration of an
aging "dynamic" with the characteristics of a general population. In essence, the fit of aging with generalized human characteristics is difficult.
As age changes, disability and the onset of memory loss occur, older
adult populations grow increasingly diverse. Special requirements require special product and environmental design. A literature that depicts
some of this change is cited as consistent with Lawton's philosophy and
research. *[Article copies available for a fee from The Haworth Document Delivery Service: 1-800-HAWORTH. E-mail address: <getinfo@haworthpressinc.com>
Website: <http://www.HaworthPress.com> © 2003 by The Haworth Press, Inc. All
rights reserved.]*

KEYWORDS. Technology and aging, micro-environment, product design, environmental design, disability

Joseph A. Koncelik is affiliated with the Center for Assistive Technology and Environmental Access, Georgia Institute of Technology.

[Haworth co-indexing entry note]: "The Human Factors of Aging and the Micro-Environment: Personal
Surroundings, Technology and Product Development." Koncelik, Joseph A. Co-published simultaneously in
Journal of Housing for the Elderly (The Haworth Press, Inc.) Vol. 17, No. 1/2, 2003, pp. 117-134; and: *Physical Environments and Aging: Critical Contributions of M. Powell Lawton to Theory and Practice* (ed: Rick J.
Scheidt, and Paul G. Windley) The Haworth Press, Inc., 2003, pp. 117-134. Single or multiple copies of this
article are available for a fee from The Haworth Document Delivery Service [1-800-HAWORTH, 9:00 a.m. -
5:00 p.m. (EST). E-mail address: getinfo@haworthpressinc.com].

M. Powell Lawton's research and insights about environment and behavior transcended both the field of gerontology and the disciplinary focus of the social sciences. His prolific writings and depth of research influenced generations of interior and industrial designers, architects, product development engineers, human factors specialists, furniture designers and many who chose to identify aging as a critical philosophic theme in their work. Lawton defined the microenvironment and demonstrated the connection between architecture, personal space and those objects everyone chooses to live with–and those we don't. It seems appropriate to establish his impact on the understanding of this connectivity by stating a basic concept central to his definition of the micro-environment as a critical component of space and surroundings–not distinct or less important than the larger architectural context of environment. Lawton (1990) noted the importance of the *control center* as an essential aspect of the micro-environment. The control center consists of a chair oriented to acquire maximum information about what he called the *near environment.*

The intent of this article is to discuss the breadth and depth of what Lawton called the micro-environment. It is important to establish context and identify criteria for designing "from the skin the walls," as the micro-environment has been colorfully described, for aging adults. This context includes those things that fill space of the personal environment including the design criteria, specification and selection of products, appliances and furnishings that must relate to and accommodate the "process" of aging.

THE SIGNIFICANCE OF THE MICRO-ENVIRONMENT

It is an interesting proposition to address the issue of interior "design" and the environmental requirements of an aging population. The residential environments of the single family dwelling unit is defined and designed by its owners. The aging population–especially the oldest among us–has a greater attachment to their personal environment than other age groups. The surroundings of the home environment takes on increasingly greater significance as people age because personal history is defined by those surroundings and they are likely to spend more of their time in their residence. Personal space and the surroundings of personal objects are important in the establishment of a sense of well-being and control.

M. Powell Lawton, as demonstrated in the previous quote, stated that personal space and control over that environment is a sign of control over one's own existence. Without that control, a sense of well-being may be lost and elderly experience real physical–as well as psychological–decline. In this complex design milieu, the designer advises–the designer may present alternatives and the designer cooperates with the older resident to insure that decisions about surroundings are made to the complete satisfaction of the aging resident. The overarching responsibility of the designer is the safety, security and sense of satisfaction of the elderly resident who, in the final analysis, must live with the designs others produce.

Sandra Howell (1976, 1978 and 1980), a colleague of M. Powell Lawton, carefully observed what the elderly prefer in their living arrangements in order to establish criteria for the development of other architectural and interior settings. Personal artifacts of choice imbue an environment with personality, reflect the lifestyle of the aging resident and, more importantly, provide the aging individual with a sense of control over environment and over their own existence. Environmental research in the late 1960s and throughout the 1970s (Kira, 1966; Pastalan and Carson, 1970; M. P. Lawton, 1975) illuminated our understanding of the differences between the environments of older adults and younger individuals. Concepts such as home range, personal space and tools such as empathic modeling informed generations of designers.

Research has demonstrated that older adults naturally acquire many things during their lifetime and seem to be living with "clutter" (Koncelik, Ostrander and Snyder, 1972). Display of personal objects: photographs, collections, assorted memorabilia and other "accessories" were and are observable in the home settings of the aged. Those older adults who have moved from one environment to another usually experience a compression of their living arrangements and belongings. In most instances, the transition from the home to something else means less space and the need to choose between things accumulated over a lifetime (Howell, 1976, 1978). Living independently in surroundings of choice with personal belongings is part of that aspect of life wherein accumulation is part of memory. Each object in the home of an older person takes on a precious quality of reminiscence. As the concept of aging in place has taken hold, understanding the relationship of environment to well-being raises in significance. Memory—and the fading of short term memory—can be attached to the familiarity of personal environment.

Aspects of very high-tech surveillance technology are being used to record behaviors during tasks performed by older adults who are experiencing the onset of memory loss. These tasks will be subject to interventions—interruptions—that will provide information about how memory, and the lack of short-term memory, allows or does not allow task continuation. Additionally, miniature cameras worn on the person will record gestures made during conversation and activities—potentially used for the creation of a system of signaling for environmental control by older adults at the onset of memory loss. An article in *Advanced Imaging* discusses the coming of commercial product systems that will image gestures made by the hands, store these images as data in a computer and use them to signal technology within the environment–light switches, VCRs, television sets, thermostats, security systems, even microwave ovens. Initial research conducted by Gandy, Starner, Ashbrook and Auxier at Georgia Tech (Lake, 2001) has produced definitions and optimization of so-called "control gestures" they hope will contribute to control of environment by older adults at the onset of memory loss.

AGING AND DISABILITY

The relationship of disability to aging is undeniable and of great importance. As population segments age beyond 75, the overwhelming number of adults will be experiencing moderate to severe disability (Todd, Deloache, and Koncelik, 1997). Acquisition of products and technology to accommodate the needs of people with disabilities also has a very strong relationship to age. Seventy-five percent of all assistive technology is acquired by older adults (Todd, Deloache, and Koncelik 1997). The issue of disability has a profound impact upon decision making regarding environment and presents issues related to continuance within an environment, the home, affecting the preferred model of living, aging in place.

Independent aging adults experiencing disability ranges from the middle-old to the old-old, approximately 15% of the population of independent aging people, depending upon how the statistical information about this population is interpreted. It is a population that is characterized by increasing heterogeneity with multiple physiological afflictions. Harrell, Eherlich and Hubbard (1990) characterize this elderly population as among "the vulnerable aged." M. Powell Lawton summarizes his conception of this population in this same text as being made up of ". . . 1.3 million in institutions, 2.5 million relatively homebound people in ordinary communities and 0.3 million in planned housing, a total of 4.1 million or about 14% of all older people."

The oldest among the American population have at least 2 chronic afflictions, typically arthritis and related muscle and bone disorders. The range of disorders include a broad based spectrum of moderate and severe disabilities from arthritis, at a disabling level, through to the onset of Alzheimer's Disease which affects marital relationships and care giving. The age segment suffering high levels of disability also has modest to low income. Their greatest asset is their home and other real properties. According to U.S. Census data (1994), of the 19.5 million households headed by an elderly person, 75% own their own homes and 25% are renters. Yet again, as reported by American Association of Retired Persons (1990), about 30% of all non-institutionalized older persons lived alone in 1989–an increase of 25% since 1980.

Accommodation of the needs of the aging with disabilities within residential environments increases in individual specialization of response (Graeff and Singer, 1988). With such high proportions of older adults living alone and, having a propensity for moderate to severe disabilities, the need for in-home health care and monitoring interventions is clearly significant especially over the next thirty years.

Human factors is a body of knowledge encompassing the characteristics, capabilities and performance of the human being meant for application to design process. Designers generally prefer a conceptual model of human factors that allows maximum application of general characteristics encompassing the broadest range of population for the development of products, interiors and architecture. Aging is a dynamic construct in the composition of human factors. Aging is difficult to blend with general human characteristics because it is continuous and occurs at different rates to different people. As a dynamic human factor, aging is a complex blending of physiological, psychophysical, psychological and sociological change. Aging is a process of change to human personality through intensification of individual characteristics. People who have reached advanced years (75-95) will be a very diverse population with increased difference between individuals than younger populations.

More that 30 years ago, Pastalan (1970) referred to normal age change as the "Age/Loss Continuum" and has application to product and environmental development. The continuum specifically pertains to sensory modality change and is the most general and widely distributed set of aging characteristics. These changes are the basis for developing products that are inclusive of both younger and older age segments as users. The onset of age related changes are the essential set of characteristics that define who is referred to as an aging adult. While it is not common to depict people in the 40 to 50 age range as aged, the progression of change defines aging.

These normal age changes affect human performance, but are not disabilities or distinctive characteristics separating aging adults from a so-called general population. James Pirkl's (1994) concept of "Transgenerational Design," is one designer's effort to demonstrate the plausibility of integration of normal age changes–separate from disabilities–with the body of human factors characteristics of the general population. As Pirkl has proposed, aging is normal and age related changes should be treated as part of the normal spectrum of human factors design criteria.

Human factors criteria that encompass the dynamic of aging begins then with changes that can be seen as general and not related to disability. Normal age change is the crucial ingredient required in an integration of characteristics that will define and determine general product and technology development.

The sensory modalities of vision, hearing, touch, taste, and smell are subject to change in varying amounts and define the aging dynamic as part of human factors.

Vision, Color and Lighting

The contemporary world with its emphasis on technology has tremendously increased the amount of information delivered visually and has also developed complex systems of signs and symbols to guide individuals through environments or to locate environments. The human eye is an edge sensitive visualization device. It is equipped to see shape and discriminate one shape from another. Animals and insects have different capabilities for visualization, some with much higher capabilities to see motion, pattern, and an extended range of the color spectrum. Human beings are able to perceive shape depending upon the color of that shape to a greater or lesser degree. The human eye has color sensitive photo pigmentation dispersed in the cones of the eye in the proportions of 64% red, 32% green and 2% blue (Murch, 1987). Blue photo pigmentation, the least prevalent, is dispersed in the cones furthest from the macula location on the retina with the highest ability to focus light. The fovea of the macula on the retina has almost complete "blue-blindness" and blue shape can frequently disappear when the eye is fixed upon them (Murch, 1987). The very center of the retina, while high in acuity, is practically devoid of blue sensitive cones. Blue-blindness is the disappearance of blue light objects when one fixates upon them. More importantly, the eye must continuously shift to "read" blue light, and thus objects in blue fatigue the eye faster than other colors. These conditions are general and not age related. However, all color sensitivity decreases with age and blue color sensitivity is gradually lost with age at varying rates of change depending upon the individual.

Color sensitivity, especially sensitivity to color transmitted in light rather than pigment, has assumed much greater significance with the development of computers and other "graphical user interfaces" or "GUIs" that proliferate among all information technologies in use today. Preference for color has little to do with accurate perception of information in color. Many individuals prefer light transmitted color combinations that cause greater fatigue to the eye and difficulty in legibility of information. With a higher number of older adults in the work force than ever before, understanding appropriate work station design that includes light transmitted information on screen surfaces is critical to continuous performance.

Other conditions of change to vision and the eye also affect perception. There is a reduction in transmittance of light through the fluid that supports the eye with age. This change affects both the perception of color and the perception of objects in light. Foveal vision (the ability to focus on edges in light) declines with age, with increases in loss of ability after the age of 40. This is directly attributable to a hardening of the lens of the eye and the inability of the muscle controllers to alter the shape of the lens to focus the light on the retina. Muscles controlling the lens weaken with age. At 50, most people begin to experience heightened sensitivity to glare as the opacity of the lens increases. This opacity also has the effect of reducing the intensity of all colors as well. The lens also begins to "yellow" with time and this has the effect of altering color perception–especially the perception of blue light. After 70, virtually 100% of the population requires the use of glasses or other prosthetic focusing device.

Adaptation to differing light levels changes with age. At age 70, the human eye adapts to changes in light levels 3 times slower than the eye at 25. This is especially important where individuals are expected to move through an environment of dramatic light changes, such as driving into a parking garage or under an overpass on a highway, or moving through a corridor with great shifts in the variance of lighting. Older people tend to slow down to accommodate to these fluctuations in lighting levels so that they are able to process information from the environment at a rate that their senses can handle (Koncelik, 1987). Other vision changes include: yellowing of the cornea, changes in the viscosity of the eye fluids causing alteration to the transmittance of all light and crazing or scratching of the cornea–further exacerbating the problem of glare.

Glare is the second most important issue to consider in the application of lighting. While three times the illumination is necessary to perform tasks, the aging eye is more highly susceptible to glare–and fatigues more quickly. There are three types of glare that concern designers and those who select and specify lighting for environments for the aging. There are three types of glare: direct, indirect and specular. Direct glare is the unnecessary and unwanted illumination form of glare from a lighting source. Indirect is reflective glare off surfaces and specular glare is the star-burst effect of light reflecting from a highly polished surface.

Lighting and color in light as it relates to human behavior is a complex topic that has been the subject of a special category of literature (Nuckolls, 1976; Birren, 1978). It is difficult to be comprehensive on the subject of lighting even with a text because the technology of lighting has been rapidly advancing over the past two decades. Just as lighting is both natural and artificial, lighting must be seen in its qualitative and quantitative forms and with regard to the color of lighting. Understanding color in light–and color sensitivity in general–is a very difficult proposition that is fraught with design mysticism and myth. *Color and Human Response* by Faber Birren (1978) is a work every designer should read before accepting closely held design credos related to environmental applications of color pigmentation and color in lighting. Birren debunks the witchcraft but, unfortunately, prejudice is far too strong a brew and, regardless of evidence to the contrary, design education and practice hold strongly to notions such as pink walls calming prisoners in a penitentiary and red lighting enhancing sales in retail outlets.

As many behavioral scientists will attest, the variables present in the physical environment are so numerous that there can be no specific determination of a predictable relationship between lighting, color and behavior. No consistent research effort has demonstrated that color on walls or color in light has a definable behavioral effect upon people. While behaviors may modify under varying environmental conditions they may either be subject to numerous interrelated variables or be only a short-term reaction to a dramatic change in an environment with which the user had already been familiar. Accommodation, adaptation and foveal vision are performance issues relating the capability of the human eye to perception under varying light conditions. Accommodation is the ability of the eye to see at different distances. Adaptation is accommodation under varying lighting conditions. Foveal vision is a reference to performance of tasks under illumination. It generally takes the aging eye at 70 years three times as long to adapt or accommodate than the human eye at 25. It takes three times as much illumination to see objects and perform tasks at 70 than at the age of 25. In other words, the aged eye is slower to respond and requires more illumination to perform.

Task illumination is that light necessary to perform various functions. This may range from reading in a static position under direct illumination or playing tennis while moving rapidly from one position in a space to another. Task illumination lighting products have improved dramatically. High output sources, today, use a fraction of the energy of sources or bulbs of the past and permit more indirect lighting in all forms in environments–even for task illumination.

Hearing

A world without sound may be much more devastating to contemplate. Sound is first and foremost a warning device to let the organism know if danger is nearby. In the modern world, those individuals who isolate themselves with in-ear radios to screen out the environment are increasing the potential hazard of a threatening environment–and doubly injurious–hastening loss of hearing. Younger populations' hearing is testing more poorly, giving rise to speculation about eventual significant levels of hearing loss among future older adults.

Hearing is also a feedback mechanism that informs us about ourselves and our own ability. Most importantly, loss of hearing affects quality of speech. In order to speak distinctly, it is necessary to hear our own speech continuously.

As hearing declines, speech is also negatively affected. Totally deaf people who have suffered trauma induced or progressive hearing loss will speak less clearly. It is necessary to undergo speech therapy with hearing loss in order to maintain this vital method of communication. This interrelationship is a critical example of how human well-being and sense of self can be determined by physiological change.

The hearing change associated with normal aging is selective frequency hearing loss, or Presbycusis. Selective frequency hearing loss has an early onset for many individuals commonly detected at the age of 40. It is a change in the ability to detect high frequency sounds. The result is an inability to discriminate between sounds such as conversation and background noise. Amplitude losses (lessening of the ability to hear low levels of "volume" of sound) in hearing are also common with aging but not inherent to the aging process. Environmental noise is playing an increasing role in debilitating a greater proportion of the hearing the loudness of sounds among all populations.

Just a few years ago, the hearing aid industry did not have technologies that would provide prostheses in hearing for anything but amplitude loss. Most hearing aids are amplitude devices at the lowest level of intervention. However, rapid technological change has increased progress toward technologies for frequency sensitivity. Micro-chip controlled miniaturized hearing aids are now available allowing for amplitude and frequency modulation of sound. Additionally, the reliability of hearing aids was poor just a few years ago, but here again the industry has sought to improve reliability and longevity of the products they manufacture and support with service. New hearing aids can either be set to amplify sounds in specific frequencies or automatically adjust to "listen" for specific frequencies. Computer controlled aids will allow the user to select hearing "channels" by pressing buttons on a microprocessor controlled remote unit. This permits the user to adjust hearing to the environment and select sounds.

Presbycusis is selective frequency hearing loss–commencing at around the age of 40 among most adults. The highest frequencies are those most susceptible to loss. This loss means that consonant sounds in speech and the discrimination of specific background environmental noises are confused. It is harder for an older person to focus upon a conversation and not have that conversation "invaded" by other sounds in the environment.

Sound attenuation in the environment is also an important consideration (Koncelik, 1987). All too frequently, the materials selected and the architecture itself amplify and mix sound that increases the problem rather than ameliorating it. While there is a technological and industry focus upon the design of improved prostheses for hearing, the interior designer has a major contribution to make by paying attention to the selection and application of materials throughout a setting that would enhance the ability of an elderly person to use it.

Physiology

Of all the various disciplines that contribute information to the body of knowledge on the human factors of aging, those disciplines such as physiology, exercise physiology and the medical related disciplines have contributed the most. David Lamb (1984) a noted exercise physiologist, demonstrated that aerobic fitness among aging adults can be improved with exercise. In his work, "aerobic endurance performance" was substantially increased through regular and carefully regulated exercise. Very recently, programs of free weight lifting among institutionalized elderly improved strength and flexibility. This and other methods of improving fitness were discounted only a short time ago. Therefore, while our knowledge base is rich, it is growing and concepts of health and fitness are changing.

There is increasing heterogeneity among the aging population, with multiple physiological afflictions, at least 2 chronic afflictions for everyone over 80–arthritis and related muscular/skeletal disorders. Michael Teague (1991) points out that *functional impairment* is loss or abnormality of physical or psychological structure or function. This means that many of the infirm aged are functionally impaired and require environmental, product and service supports. Teague describes physiological change that occurs to individuals as "psychomotor aging." According to Teague, normal age changes occur including changes to the nervous system, cardiopulmonary system, and the muscular-skeletal system. Muscle mass declines by approximately 40% by the age of 70. Losses in strength are specific and especially severe in the quadriceps (40%) and in the arm muscles.

These changes have important ramifications for the design of environments as well as products such as chairs and other furnishings. Obviously, characteristic losses in strength and flexibility will mean less ability to negotiate complex environments that are not designed with consideration for those aging adults in advanced years who have experienced losses in physical capability. With regard to the products that make up the micro environment, transferring weight successfully and lifting away from a chair becomes significantly more difficult after the age of 70. Flexibility and closure of the joints in the extremities is also decreased. Knee closure combined with losses in strength mean that the foot cannot be moved rearward under the center of gravity of the body as easily.

AGING AND TECHNOLOGY

Time of day is also an important consideration regarding the ebb and flow of strength and flexibility among the elderly. Frequently, older people are beset with tremor in their hands and reduced strength to perform tasks in the early morning and in the evening. Bending over is difficult, generally speaking, and may result in dizziness and fainting at times.

In order for the human factors information to have meaning it is necessary to extrapolate principals derived from research and extended through the experience of application. Some deductions about the application of physiological and psychological human performance to environment and technology have been set out in the literature. This literature is exemplified by Byerts and Koncelik (1976), Pastalan (1970), and Lawton (1975). During this period, Byerts and Lawton produced the literature on environment and behavior that explored guidelines that have been applied in architecture and in product development. These guidelines for application of visual signals and cues would include: *Redundant Cueing*–use more than one sensory modality to "signal" the aging user. Combine visual cues with sound cues or visual cues with tactile cues to increase the "legibility" of devices. Redundancy of cues can also back up the cue in one sensory modality with another cue using that same modality to increase the "legibility" of devices. A color may be supported by a pictogram or a "beep" sound cue followed by a voice cue. *Color coding* has been overestimated in its value because the meaning of the code is not always clear or the colors visible in the specific illumination of a particular environment cannot be clearly seen. Additionally, complex color codes in environments can be more confusing than helpful.

The essence of "human factors" is its capacity for application to design of environments and products. In appliance design, issues of aging are intertwined with marketing to more than one age segment. Appliance products will tend to be less specialized and selection becomes critical. High technology applications require that attention to issues of age change to sensory modalities to insure appropriate control and display design.

For over two decades, significant interest has been generated in the relationship of accident to age. In a report utilizing the data base from the U.S. Consumer Product Safety Commission, Czaja and Drury (1982) developed a human factors model of accident occurrence to explain the higher rate of accidents among older adults. The authors define the model as accident occurrence when there exists a "mismatch" between the demands of a task (or the environment) and the capabilities of the "operator." An earlier study of tasks in bathing and food preparation by Drury and Brill (1983) produced the conclusion that the "momentary" demands of the task may exceed the "momentary" capabilities of the person. It is possible then for any person, regardless of age, to be presented with a situation in the home that will provide demands that will make the possibility of accident higher. For the elderly, with diminished sensory and physiological capability, the demands need not be an overload situation and the threshold of accident proneness crossed rather easily.

The problem of accidents among the elderly is a substantial one. Accidents rank fifth among all causes of death for people over the age of 65 (Czaja, Drury, Hammond, Brill and Lofti, 1982). The elderly suffer a higher rate of death due to accidents than do younger age segments in the population and also suffer a higher degree of injury as a result of accidents. The statistical evidence with regard to specific accidents, number of elderly and types of causes is prodigious with approximately 25 thousand deaths every year for people over the age of 65 and nearly a million injuries. The cost to the nation in terms of personal loss as well as financial loss is too high when both home modifications and detection technologies are currently available that could ameliorate the problem. In the BOSTI study (Czaja et al., 1982) it was found that 43% of all accidents in the home involved people over the age of 65. Fire related accidents are the most severe in terms of human lives lost, injuries and property and financial losses. Accidents related to smoking are still among the leading reasons for fire in the home. Elderly also have more accident problems with products and appliances than any other age group. The leading product category that produces accidents among the elderly is floor and flooring materials according to the BOSTI study that extended outward to include such hazardous products as ladders and lawn mowers.

The *bathroom, kitchen, bedroom* are the most critical spaces within the residence, and living space is significant as central to control of the personal environment for every person. These spaces intensify in importance for aging adults. Of significance is one fact that has been mentioned earlier: there has been little change in the environment among housing units owned by the middle-old and old-old independent infirm aged in the United States. Most of these housing units have had little change. If any change has occurred, it is likely that the aged person has made that change. Typically such change would include the addition of a grab bar on the wall or the tub in the bathroom or modifications to storage in the kitchen. Since entrance and egress from the home is a fundamental consideration, the addition of a ramp from the front or back door is an easy modification in most instances. Independence is supported or impeded by accessibility (Pynoos, Cohen, Davis, and Bernhardt, 1987).

Designing new bathrooms within an architectural design project and refurbishing older bathrooms are very complex tasks that would include numerous points for consideration. In refurbishing older bathroom facilities, if the interior walls and overall plan affords an option to do so, the most significant modification to the bathroom would be to increase the size of the bathroom door and change the swing of the door from inward to outward. It has been something of a misanthropic design convention to place 26 inch wide bathroom doors in homes–and this convention persists even in modern home building today. In the design of new facilities, wheelchair access to toilets must follow wheelchair access through the door to the bathroom. Most wheelchairs are approximately 27 inches wide and the minimum door should be no less than 30 inches wide. If the residence to be built is to be designed from the ground up, a 32 inch doorway into the bathroom is a minimum standard to be observed.

As an important safety measure, a telephone should be installed in the bathroom. Older people who live alone are more susceptible to falls in this area of the home than any other. Access to the phone must be carefully considered from a prone position or technological features employed that will allow phone access without physical contact. New construction permits consideration of numerous technological alternatives to this problem. Bathroom design is changing and recognition of the issues of aging will help to serve a greater range of users from those who have no physical problems to those who may be either moderately or severely disabled.

The most significant aspect of the design of kitchens to accommodate aging adults is understanding the changes in food preparation and food preference that occur over time. Large meals with large quantities of food served in three distinct meals fade from preference–especially among those elderly who live alone. Smaller meals are preferred or what can be termed a continuous eating pattern throughout the day without a specific meal preparation. There are more convenience foods utilized and less oven use for baking and other long term cooking. The microwave oven and other convenience table-top cooking devices are preferred over the large appliance cooker that requires more complex operations–and bending and stretching movements difficult for an older person. The quantity of foods requiring refrigeration declines and space devoted to large stand-alone refrigerators may be wasted space. Smaller refrigerators in the four cubic feet size should be explored for selection. A version that is counter top rather than under-counter in design would be preferred.

In appliance design and product selection, high technology requires that attention be placed upon appropriate control and display design. The designer must understand age related changes to sensory modalities–vision and hearing–in order to design consumer sensitive products. Vanderheiden and Vanderheiden (1991) have taken a somewhat different approach to the design of controls and displays by defining "accessibility" as both a physiological and psychological operational task. In their work, resulting design configurations result from how elderly respond to various controls and displays as much as through physiological criteria.

One of the progressive changes in the use of standard kitchen arrangements is the gradual disuse of storage above and below the waist level or counter top. First, fewer foodstuffs are present in the kitchen of an older person. Second, whatever has been purchased may be more accessible and provide memory cues when things are visible.

Parsons (1972) was one a pioneer on human factors research on the bedroom. The bedroom is a locus of daily living activities and a focus for complex human behaviors. The primary behavior that gives rise to any space designated as a bedroom is, of course, sleeping. However, sleeping in and of itself is a complex behavior that is only just beginning to be understood in relationship to aging. Generally, older adults sleep less (some research states that older people require less sleep). They also do not achieve the deep sleep of younger people which is a disadvantage in terms of total restfulness and an advantage with regard to emergency warning of the elderly when there may be life threatening circumstances such as fire. Sleeping becomes less confined to the bedroom for older adults. They may move about during the night and choose other places within the residence to sleep. The bedroom remains the central focus for resting and sleeping and frequently becomes the point of departure for restless waking and selection of alternative sleep space.

The frequency of visitation to the bathroom increases with age and thus the location of these two critical components of the interior must be seen as proximate. While this is less of a problem in new construction, the design of older homes generally owned by the very old have fewer bathrooms and they can be more distant from the bedroom than in new construction. Renovation projects may require study of the alternative to build new bathroom facilities externally attached to the home or consider products and appliances that can be placed in the bedroom.

The bedroom is another appropriate location for a telephone. The telephone is an important first line of support for safety and security enabling direct access to the outside world. The need for general communications is augmented by the need for support in times of illness and injury. The American Association of Retired Persons reported in 1990 that two thirds of all elderly who have living children live within thirty minutes traveling time from a child. Sixty-two percent of those elderly persons have visitations from a child on a weekly basis and 76% talk weekly on a telephone to their children.

Living-room space for the older adult will have a control center (Lawton, 1990). A chair positioned to allow the older person to access visually, and audibly, any and all significant areas of the home will anchor a control center. This will include the front door and a view through a window to the entrance or approach to the home and the kitchen area. The control center should be proximate to a telephone. It should also provide for activities of personal preference such as reading and writing and activities such as hobbies or long-term personal interests.

The living space in the compressed living arrangements of the apartment or small home will also become a primary display area of those collectibles and memorabilia that identify place and control of the environment by the elderly occupant. Shelving and storage units are important considerations as well as the provision of wall surface for the display of photographs or other personal decorative items.

The human performance and preference issue that is significant regarding environmental conditioning and control is that of temperature. Older people prefer warmer temperatures and feel colder faster than do younger adults. It is important to keep in mind, however, that older people fatigue more easily in high heat when performing tasks. Central air conditioning, both in terms of temperature and with regard to air filtration, is a commonplace technology in contemporary heating, ventilating and air conditioning systems (HVAC). Home monitoring systems (HMS), including technology for safety and security, are technologies that are rapidly changing and becoming integrated as a single centrally controlled home system. Security systems can survey the residence and signal the approach of visitors. These multifunctional devices may also monitor vital signs. Through lighting can be controlled and timed, emergency conditions such as fire and hazardous emissions monitored, located and signaled, and routine maintenance of the home continuously monitored and communicated.

Computers are now a commonplace product technology in the home environment. Older adults use computers–and have some age-related problems with their use. In his book about the complexity of computer operations, Raskin (2000) coined the term "double-dysclicksia" and discusses the problem of having someone double-click on a file or computer icon in order to open or access the file or program. Double clicking requires of the user the ability to hold the cursor steady and click twice within .125 seconds. This is the standard or norm for computer operations and it is undoable for many older people. There are accessibility remedies in most PC and MacIntosh operating systems–if the user is aware of them. One can experience the difficulty by using a computer mouse with the opposite hand from which one normally interacts with the computer. Holding a cursor steady and clicking within the allotted time is not a trivial matter–considering how often computer users do this every day. Software is now available to allow communication between a home computer and other appliances–permitting signaling of kitchen ranges left on, interior climate controls that the home owner can talk to and even communication from the computer about the timing of medications. New surface scanning technologies not only provide clothing manufacturers to fit everyone perfectly with mass-customized garments; the same technology can be used to gather body images relevant to health and well-being. In my center, we are currently using full-body scanning to gather a new database on the body measurements of older adults. There are commercial organizations developing home health care strategies that employ computer monitoring and control to provide care to older adults.

Every computer can be specified and acquired with variable forms of interface for the aging user. Many new machines come equipped with "accessibility" software for the modification of interfaces as standard equipment. The amount of information to be tracked and processed is increasing at a time for some when their capacity to understand, access and process such information is declining. In order to offset this problem, the designer must pay attention to the rate of information flow, the limitations of perception that come with normal age losses and such principals as redundant cueing to insure that signals and communications are received and can be processed. Many design changes are being made to address problems with the use of computer technology by older adults and individuals with disabilities. Synthesized voice reminders, repeated and redundantly signaled messages in verbal and sound output are used to ward off the problem of confusion about drug dosage, time of dosage and rate of administration.

CONCLUSIONS

Age changes affect understanding and design of the micro-environment in profound ways. Of the greatest concern in residential design is sustaining the independence of that population who is "vulnerable." Aging in place, as a concept, requires a different approach from design professions. How designers address issues of aging begins with education–reeducation if necessary. The vulnerability of the independent aging living with moderate to severe levels of disability cannot always be accomplished by amalgamating their characteristics with the general population. The problems of designing for the oldest Americans require an understanding of their diversity.

The vast body of information about older adults should serve to inform designers that mass marketing concepts and efforts to homogenize the aging population into a single market segment will fail. Older adults with disabilities require special product development and special marketing techniques while product and environmental designs that are developed for the general population may well serve the young-old.

Designing for older people requires humility on the part of the designer; a willingness to release closely held ideas about designing for its own sake in order to serve a greater purpose. In that regard, M. Powell Lawton and other gerontologists have provided a significant lesson for all designers–regardless of whether or not that lesson is immediately perceived. Older adults inform us about their requirements and as their numbers grow, so will their impact upon residential environmental design as well as the design and marketing of consumer products. Observing and listening to what they say and show us is a requirement, not an option.

REFERENCES

American Association of Retired Persons. (1990). *A profile of older Americans.* (EE-0107) Washington, D.C. 1990.

Birren, F. (1978). *Color and human response.* New York: Van Nostrand Reinhold Publishers.

Byerts, T. O., & Koncelik, J.A. (1976). (Eds.) *Designing housing products for the elderly and the handicapped.* Proceedings of a Gerontological Society Conference. Washington, D.C.

Czaja, S. J., Drury, C., Hammond, K., Brill, M. & Lofti, V. (1982). *Aging and accidents with consumer products: The size and nature of the problem.* A Report to the Administration on Aging: Buffalo, NY: The Buffalo Organization for Social and Technological Innovation, University of New York at Buffalo.

Czaja, Sara J., & Drury, C. (1982). *Patterns of consumer product accidents.* A Report to the Administration on Aging: Buffalo, NY: The Buffalo Organization for Social and Technological Innovation, University of New York at Buffalo.

Drury, C.G. & Brill, M. (1983). Human factors in consumer product accident investigation. *Human Factors,* 25, 329-343.

Graeff, R. F. & Singer, L. (1988). *A bathroom for the elderly: Aging factors, design evaluation criteria and a design proposal.* Blacksburg, Virginia: Center for Product and Environmental Design, Virginia Polytechnic Institute.

Harrell, Z., Ehrlich, P. & Hubbard, R. (1990). (Eds.). *The vulnerable aged: People, services and policies.* New York: Springer Publishing Company.

Howell, S. T. (1976). *Shared spaces in housing for the elderly.* Cambridge, Massachusetts: Institute of Technology Press.

Howell, S. T. (1978). Aging and social leaning of a new environment. In H. O. K. Shimada (Ed.), *Recent Advances in Gerontology: Proceedings of the XI International Congress of Gerontology,* Tokyo, Japan, International Congress of Gerontology Series Number 469, pp. 371-376.

Howell, S. T. (1980). *Designing for aging: Patterns of use.* Cambridge, Massachusetts: The MIT Press.

Kira, A. (1966). *The bathroom.* New York: Viking Press.

Koncelik, J. A., Ostrander, E., & Snyder, L.H. (1972). *The new nursing home: Conference proceedings.* Ithaca, New York: Cornell University.

Koncelik, J. A. (1987). Product and furniture design for the chronically impaired elderly. In V. Regnier & J. Pynoos (Eds.), *Housing the aged: Design directives and public policy* (pp. 373-398). New York: Elsevier Science Publishing Company.

Lake, D. (2001). Gesture recognition for the consumer: Helping the elderly retain control of their world. *Advanced Imaging Magazine*, 16, 5, 34-36.

Lamb, D. R. (1984). *Physiology of exercise: Responses and adaptations*. New York: Macmillan Publishing.

Lawton, M. P. (1975). *Planning and managing housing for the elderly*. New York: John Wiley and Sons.

Lawton, M. P. (1990). Vulnerability and socioenvironmental factors. In Z. Harrel, P. Ehrlich, & R. Hubbard (Eds.), *The vulnerable aged: People, services, and policies* (pp. 104-115). New York: Springer Publishing Company.

Murch, G. (1987). Human factors of displays. In *Colors in Computer Graphics: Course Notes*. Los Angeles: Siggraph Conference.

Nuckolls, J. L. (1976). *Interior lighting for environmental designers*. New York: John Wiley and Sons.

Parsons, H. M. (1972). The bedroom. *Human Factors*, 14 (5), 421-450.

Pastalan, L.A. (1970). Privacy as an expression of human territoriality. In L. A. Pastalan & D. Carson (Eds.), *Spatial behavior of older people* (pp. 88-101). Ann Arbor, MI: University of Michigan Press.

Pirkl, J. (1994). *Transgenerational design: Designing products for an aging population*. New York: Van Nostrand Reinhold.

Pynoos, J., Cohen, E., Davis, L., & Bemhardt, S. (1987). Home modifications: Improvements that extend independence. In V. Regnier & J. Pynoos (Eds.), *Housing the aged: Design directives and public policy* (pp. 277-303). New York: Elsevier Science Publishing.

Raskin, J. (2000). *The humane interface: New directions for designing interactive systems*. Reading, MA: Addison-Wesley Publishers.

Teague, M. A. (1991). Leisure product development: Outlining the need. In *Independent living environments for seniors and persons with disabilities: Proceedings and directions '91*. The Canadian Aging and Rehabilitation Product Development Corporation. Winnipeg, Manitoba, Canada.

Todd, R., DeLoache, S., & Koncelik, J. A. (1997). *Disabilities category and marketing matrix*. A report for the Center for Rehabilitation Technology, Georgia Institute of Technology, Atlanta, Georgia.

U. S. Bureau of the Census (1994). *Statistical abstracts of the United States*, U.S. Department of Commerce (114th. Edition). Washington, D.C: U.S. Government Printing Office.

Vanderheiden, G.C., & Vanderheiden, K.R. (1991). *Accessible design of consumer products*. A Report for the AD-HOC Industry-Consumer-Researcher Work Group of the Consumer Product Design Guidelines Project, Department of Industrial Engineering, University of Wisconsin-Madison.

Toward Measuring Proactivity in Person-Environment Transactions in Late Adulthood: The Housing-Related Control Beliefs Questionnaire

Frank Oswald
Hans-Werner Wahl
Mike Martin
Heidrun Mollenkopf

SUMMARY. Both a life-span developmental control perspective as well as an environmental gerontology view, particularly Lawton's notion of environmental proactivity, served as the theoretical background to suggest a new dimension of domain-specific control, namely hous-

Frank Oswald, Hans-Werner Wahl, Mike Martin, and Heidrun Mollenkopf are affiliated with The German Centre for Research on Ageing, University of Heidelberg.

Address correspondence to: Dr. Frank Oswald, The German Centre for Research on Ageing at the University of Heidelberg, Bergheimer Strasse 20, 69115 Heidelberg, Germany (E-mail: oswald@dzfa.uni-heidelberg.de).

The authors greatly appreciate the helpful comments of Elaine Wethington on an earlier draft of this manuscript.

The collection of part of the data used in this work was supported by the German Federal Ministry of Family, Senior Citizens, Women and Youth (BMFSFJ) and the Baden-Württemberg Ministry of Science, Research and Art (MWK) grant Ref. 314-1722-102/16.

[Haworth co-indexing entry note]: "Toward Measuring Proactivity in Person-Environment Transactions in Late Adulthood: The Housing-Related Control Beliefs Questionnaire." Oswald, Frank et al. Co-published simultaneously in *Journal of Housing for the Elderly* (The Haworth Press, Inc.) Vol. 17, No. 1/2, 2003, pp. 135-152; and: *Physical Environments and Aging: Critical Contributions of M. Powell Lawton to Theory and Practice* (ed: Rick J. Scheidt, and Paul G. Windley) The Haworth Press, Inc., 2003, pp. 135-152. Single or multiple copies of this article are available for a fee from The Haworth Document Delivery Service [1-800-HAWORTH, 9:00 a.m. - 5:00 p.m. (EST). E-mail address: getinfo@haworthpressinc.com].

ing-related control beliefs. The newly developed 23-item Housing-Related Control Beliefs Questionnaire (HCQ) is based on the widely used dimensions of Internal Control, External Control: Powerful Others, and External Control: Chance. In two studies of older adults ($N= 485$; 66-69 years and $N= 107$; 65-91 years), we examined the psychometric quality of the questionnaire and explored its relation with socio-structural variables, general control beliefs, and a set of housing-related aspects. Psychometric results indicate satisfactory levels of internal consistency and retest stability in all three scales of the instrument and factor analysis supported the theoretically expected three-factor solution. Also, HCQ's external control subscales were correlated with higher age, lower education, and lower income and the correlational pattern between the HCQ and a general control measure was substantial and consistent with theoretical expectations. Relations between the HCQ and objective and subjective housing-related variables tended to be low in size. These preliminary findings suggest the potential usefulness of the HCQ as a measure to address environmental proactivity in late adulthood. *[Article copies available for a fee from The Haworth Document Delivery Service: 1-800-HAWORTH. E-mail address: <getinfo@haworthpressinc.com> Website: <http://www.HaworthPress.com> © 2003 by The Haworth Press, Inc. All rights reserved.]*

KEYWORDS. Psychological control, housing-related control beliefs

Control beliefs have long been identified as important contributors to psychological well-being and successful aging in general (Abeles, 1991; Baltes & Baltes, 1986; Bandura, 1995; Lachman, 1993; Schulz & Heckhausen, 1997; Seligman, 1991). They are also of central importance for the achievement and maintenance of independence and autonomy well into old age (Reich & Zautra, 1990; Skinner, 1995). In addition, across the life-span, control beliefs become increasingly important for both coping with everyday stress and with key transitions (Brandtstädter & Renner, 1990; Moen & Wethington, 1999). However, although general control beliefs are good predictors of omnibus measures of quality of life, they tend to be less useful to predict how people cope with stressors and challenges in particular domains of everyday life (Lachman, 1986). Furthermore, life-span trajectories of control might be quite different when domain-specificity is taken into consideration. For example, age-related increases exist for overall control over work, control over finances, and control over marriage, whereas decreases exist for control over relationships with children, and control over one's sex life (Lachman & Weaver, 1998). Results from cross-sectional and longitudinal studies on domain-specific control beliefs in the domains of health and intellectual functioning suggest stable internal control beliefs and increasing external control beliefs as people age, while no consistent relationship with gender has been reported (Clark-Plaskie & Lachman, 1999; Lachman, Ziff, & Spiro, 1994).

In terms of the context in which aging takes place, the private home becomes increasingly central to everyday life as people age. Findings from research on leisure time activities and from studies on the everyday lives of the elderly suggest a reduction of the action range, especially in very old age (Moss & Lawton, 1982). Older people spend more time at home than do younger people, particularly when they suffer from competence losses. According to data from the Berlin Aging Study (BASE), about 80% of the activities of daily living take place at home (Baltes, Maas, Wilms, Borchelt, & Little, 1999). However, the home environment has strangely been neglected in current research efforts to develop an essential set of domain-specific measurement devices. Given the triad that: (1) "establishing satisfactory physical living arrangements" is a major developmental task in old age (Havighurst, 1972, p. 113); (2) staying put is among the highest personal priorities of older people (Lawton, 1985; Scheidt, 1998); and (3) striving for control has advantages for all species capable of influencing their environments (Schulz & Heckhausen, 1999), examining age-related differences and changes in housing-related control beliefs will improve our understanding of the mechanisms underlying the achievement and maintenance of autonomy and well-being in old age.

From the perspective of environmental gerontology, highlighting housing-related control beliefs in later adulthood may offer critical theoretical potential as well, providing a major conceptual link between the (physical) environment and the aging person. Housing has traditionally been addressed within environmental gerontology as a major example of the environmental impact on aging (e.g., Parmelee & Lawton, 1990; Wahl, 2001). From this perspective, a good fit between a person's needs and competencies and the environmental conditions and amenities at home is a particularly important challenge as people age (Carp & Carp, 1984; Lawton, 1999). However, most research in the field focuses primarily on the role of environmental conditions, such as objective housing amenities, and on the potential to modify the environment to help older people to stay put and to live independently as long as possible (e.g., Lanspery & Hyde, 1997; Pynoos, 1995; Steinfeld & Danford, 1999). This focus on the environmental component of person-environment transactions neglects to some extent the fact that persons themselves can be agents in modifying environments in order to live independently. Powell

Lawton has put major emphasis on this basic insight for a "good" life in old age, by adding the concept of environmental proactivity to his model of environmental docility (Lawton, 1983, 1989a).

> This hypothesis suggests that the greater the competence of the person, the more likely the person's needs and preferences will be successfully exercised to search the environment for resources to satisfy the needs (. . .). In fact, the essence of a proactively created environment is its dynamic, temporally changing quality and its inability to be separated from the user. Examples of such transactional environmental resources are the cognitive map, the perceived or cognitively organized environment, the local amenities that are used, the state of maintenance of a home, the way it is furnished (. . .) and so on. (Lawton, 1989a, p. 18f)

A good fit between the environment and the individual cannot thus be guaranteed by a flexible or supportive environment alone. Instead, it is also important to acknowledge the role of proactive attitudes of the individual towards the environment, seen from a personality point of view (Lawton, 1998; Slangen-de Kort, 1999). The construct of housing-related control beliefs to use Lawton's (1987) terms, intends to directly address this specific agency of older adults to deal with environmental press and richness, and might thus further qualify and extend the available literature on environmental control (e.g., Schulz & Brenner, 1977, Slangen-de Kort, Midden, & Wagenberg, 1998; Timko & Moss, 1989). Thus, housing-related control beliefs are regarded as a component of environmental proactivity. Obviously, however, such a construct should always be embedded within socio-structural (such as education and income) and personality-related variables, impacting on and driving person-environment relations in the housing domain in all ages (e.g., Schaie, Wahl, Mollenkopf, & Oswald, in press).

In sum, both a life-span developmental and an environmental gerontology perspective suggest a growing importance of control beliefs in everyday domains in general and in the domain of housing in particular, as people age. Therefore, the first goal of this work was to develop an instrument aimed to measure housing-related control beliefs, entitled the Housing-Related Control Beliefs Questionnaire (HCQ), and to provide first data on its psychometric properties. Drawing from earlier discussions on the need to consider the multidimensionality of control beliefs (Lachman, 1986; Levenson, 1981), the construction was based on the well-established and most commonly used dimensions of Internal Control, External Control: Powerful Others, and External Control: Chance. Due to the preliminary character of the scale construction and the psychometric results, we regard this instrument as it currently stands as *a pilot version*, subject to further testing and improvement. Our second goal was nevertheless to present these first data which empirically anchor the construct of housing-related control beliefs within a network of variables and constructs targeting socio-structural, personality-related, and housing environment-related aspects.

METHOD

Samples

Sample A. Participants in sample A were older adults from the Interdisciplinary Longitudinal Study on Adult Development (ILSE) (Martin, Ettrich, Lehr, Roether, Martin, & Fischer-Cyrulies, 2000). The ILSE is a multi-center study on adult development whose basic aim is to identify predictors of successful aging. The study assesses a wide range of data, including demographics, health, functional capacity, cognition, personality, coping behavior, and housing. Following the assumption that housing becomes a more important part of everyday life after retirement, we focused on adults from the birth cohort 1930-32 (66-69 years). This "young old" group of adults was selected assuming that they are challenged to consider retirement-related housing decisions or changes. The sample consists of $N = 485$ community-dwelling participants who attended the second measurement point of ILSE, in which the HCQ was only ready for use. Half of the participants were from East Germany (55.1%), half from West Germany (44.9%). About half of the participants were women (48.2%), about one quarter (26.2%) were living alone, and three quarters (73.8%) were living together with someone else in the same household, usually the spouse. Their subjective health status was, on average, good to satisfactory. Only some participants suffered from competence losses ($M = 2.6$; $SD = 0.8$ from 1 = "very good" to 6 = "very bad"), and average education level was 9.9 years of formal schooling ($SD = 2.3$).

Sample B. In order to have a wider age range available than in Sample A as well as to check for retest reliability, we used the HCQ in another sample of $N = 107$ community-dwelling older adults (65-91 years old; $M = 71.6$, $SD = 5.9$ years). Participants were recruited through newspaper announcements. About one half of the sample was living alone (46.7%), the other half was living together with others in the same household (53.3%), typically their spouse. There were slightly more women than men in the sample (56.1% women). Their subjective health was, on average, good to satisfactory, and relatively few participants suffered from competence losses ($M = 2.4$, $SD = 0.8$). Retest reliability was assessed after four weeks with a subgroup (N = 39) of randomly selected men and women (36.4%).

Instruments

Construction of the HCQ and its application. The challenge in creating the HCQ was to generate items that measure control beliefs, and, specifically, to adjust the wording to indicate domain-specificity, i.e., the domain of housing. Thus, various attributes of the immediate residential environment as suggested in the literature were taken into account, including housing-related instrumental and social support, stimulation within the apartment and in the immediate surrounding, as well as maintaining housing routines and habits within a familiar socio-physical environment (Lawton, 1989b, 1999; Wahl, 2001). Based upon both findings on functions of residential environments as well as on control beliefs in other life domains, 24 statements (later reduced to 23 items, see "results" section) reflecting housing-related control beliefs were generated. Item formulations were based on the dimensions "Internal Control" (IC: 8 items, for example: "In my apartment/house, everything is going to stay just as it is for I do not care what anybody says."), "External Control: Powerful Others" (ECPO: 8 items, for example: "I rely to a great extent upon the advice of others when it comes to helpful improvements to my apartment/house."), and "External Control: Chance" (ECC: 8 items, for example: "You just have to live with the way your apartment/house is; you cannot do anything about it."). Items were assessed on a five-point rating scale with higher scores reflecting higher amounts of perceived control from 1 = "not at all" to 5 = "very much."

Additional variables with potential importance for housing-related control beliefs. In terms of socio-structural variables (in addition to age and gender), the degree of education (scale from 0-5, with higher scores indicating higher degrees of education) and household income (scale from 1-11, with higher scores indicating higher income) were taken into consideration.

With respect to personality aspects, general control beliefs obviously were of particular interest. Thus, all participants were given the 14-item scale on general control beliefs from the Berlin Aging Study (BASE) (Smith, Marsiske, & Maier, 1996; Baltes, Freund, & Horgas, 1999). This scale consists of four subscales, namely "Internal control for desired events" (3 items), "Internal control for undesirable events" (3 items), "External control–Powerful others" (4 items), and "External control–Chance" (4 items). Participants have to respond using a five-point scale from 1 = "not at all" to 5 = "very much." For the purpose of this study, both internal subscales were merged into one scale in order to achieve comparability with the control dimensions used in the HCQ.

On the level of environment-related variables, housing tenure (owner vs. tenant) and selected aspects of the objective physical layout were considered. With respect to the latter, the available amount of space per person in square meters, the number of barrier-free amenities at home (summary score of nine aspects, such as wireless phone, handgrips in bathroom and toilet, separate access to the shower, options to sit down in the bathroom and when cooking, height adjustable bed) the overall lighting conditions of the home (summary score of lighting conditions in five different places at home, i.e., entrance, staircase, kitchen, bathroom, and bedroom) and a general ranking of the objective quality of the home (5-point Likert-type rating, higher scores indicating better objective standard) were used for the analyses of the present work. In addition, the following subjective environmental perceptions were assessed: Perceived housing problems (5-point Likert-type scales, higher scores indicate more perceived housing problems) and satisfaction with housing (5-point Likert-type scales, higher scores indicate higher satisfaction). Finally, place attachment to the home environment was rated by the interviewers on a five-point Likert scale from 1 = "very low" to 5 = "very high," and the perceived neighborhood safety was assessed (4-point Likert-type scales, higher scores indicating higher safety), as an indicator for the experience of the immediate outdoor environment. These ratings were based on the in-depth parts of the interview, including descriptions of everyday life or answers to the question "What makes your house a home?" Two independent raters agreed on 91.9% of the judgements (range 90.7%-93.0%) in an inter-rater reliability test covering 20% of the whole data material.

Procedure. In Sample A, a paper and pencil version of the HCQ was presented (duration about 10 minutes) within a larger set of questionnaires to each participant separately. Data-collection took place in the German Centre for Research on Aging. A trained interviewer introduced the questionnaire and was present during the examination to answer questions. Presentation of the HCQ in Sample B was identical, except that the instrument was this time applied in small groups of 8-15 persons.

RESULTS

Psychometric Properties of the HCQ

The complete list of items used in the pilot version of the HCQ is displayed in Table 1 based on Sample A data. On the descriptive data analysis level, a tendency toward higher scores across the IC items as compared with both external control item sets was observed. Nevertheless sufficient variation was available with respect to each of the dimensions as revealed by standard deviations as well as the full use of the 5-point scale in case of each item.

Next, we examined the psychometric properties of the HCQ. After examining scale consistencies, one item (Item 10: "It is up to me to keep myself informed about new developments regarding age-friendly homes and home modification") was removed from the Internal Control scale in order to improve scale consistency. Thus, further analyses are based on 23 items in total. Final internal consistencies of the three subscales varied to some degree between both samples with Cronbach's $\alpha = .59$ (A) and .68 (B) (7 IC items), $\alpha = .66$ (A) and .72 (B) (8 ECPO items), and $\alpha = .83$ (A) and .76 (B) (8 ECC items). These sizes are comparable to the ones reported of the original Levenson general control beliefs scale (Levenson, 1973, with IC $\alpha = .51$, ECPO $\alpha = .73$, ECC $\alpha = .73$), in which also a tendency toward somewhat higher alphas in both external scales was observed.

To verify the stability of the questionnaire, data from Sample B were used to assess retest reliability of the subscales within a sample of $N = 107$ older adults and based on a four-week interval. Test-retest coefficients displayed a high to medium amount of stability across four weeks (sum scores), $r_{tt \, (IC, \, 7 \, items)} = .70, p < .001, r_{tt \, (ECPO, \, 8 \, items)} = .78, p < .001$, and $r_{tt \, (ECC, \, 8 \, items)} = .50, p < .001$.

To test for the empirical dimensionality of the HCQ, we conducted a factor analysis only with the larger sample of $N = 485$ (Sample A) to determine the underlying factor structure of the 23 items of the questionnaire. The analysis using the maximum-likelihood procedure and an oblique rotation method revealed a stable three-factor solution, explaining 37.8% of the variance. All items addressing IC and ECC had highest loadings (all > .50, with one exception: Item 13: .46) on the expected factors, while four of the eight items addressing ECPO tended to load substantially on ECPO as well. As was expected, items from the External Control subscales revealed high factor loadings on both External Control factors, ECC and ECPO. The selected rotation method of the factors does not assume complete independence between the factors; rather, it allows one to examine the correlations between the factors. Based on findings from other studies (Lachman, Ziff, & Spiro, 1994; Clark-Plaskie & Lachman, 1999) and theoretical assumptions behind the scale construction, we expected the two External Control scales to be related, but neither ECC nor ECPO to be positively related to IC. There was no significant correlation between ECPO and the IC, $r_{(ECPO \times IC)} = .00$, and a small negative correlation between ECC and the IC, $r_{(ECC \times IC)} = -.11, p < .05.$, while the two External factors were positively correlated, $r_{(ECC \times ECPO)} = .24, p < .01$. Thus, our results basically confirm the assumption of three factors of housing-related control beliefs, although the need for further improvement of items and testing

TABLE 1. Means and Standard Deviations of Housing-Related Control Beliefs Questionnaire (HCQ) Items

Item (numbers in order of presentation in the questionnaire)	Mean	SD	Range
Internal control:			
1. I am able to set up my apartment/house in accordance with my own personal tastes and ideas.	4.34	0.80	1-5
4. It is up to me whether or not I make use of nearby support services and community facilities that could make my life easier.	4.21	0.87	1-5
7. In my apartment/house, everything is going to stay just as it is for I do not care what anybody says.	3.53	1.15	1-5
10. It is up to me to keep myself informed about new developments regarding age-friendly homes and home modification.	3.07	1.34	1-5
13. It is up to me whether or not I attend cultural events in my area or visit beautiful sections of my neighborhood.	4.40	0.79	1-5
16. I could not possibly trade the neighborhood I live in for another.	3.65	1.26	1-5
19. It is up to me who helps me in or around my apartment/house.	4.25	0.90	1-5
22. I am able to set up my apartment/house in accordance with my own personal tastes and ideas.	3.16	1.35	1-5
External control: Powerful other:			
2. I rely to a great extent upon the advice of *others* when it comes to helpful improvements to my apartment/house.	2.42	0.97	1-5
5. Whether or not I will be able to stay in my apartment/house will probably depend on *other persons.*	2.14	1.20	1-5
8. In order to do anything interesting or nice outside of my apartment/house, I must rely on *others.*	1.69	0.92	1-5
11. I feel myself to be dependent upon *others* in order to use the support services and community facilities in my area.	1.38	0.95	1-5
14. When *other persons* offer to help me (e.g., with housekeeping) in or around the apartment/house, I cannot say no.	2.59	1.05	1-5
17. *Others* have told me how to arrange furnishing in my apartment/house.	1.35	0.62	1-5
20. I listen to the advice of *others* when they tell me not to change anything in my apartment/house.	1.64	0.85	1-5
23. *Other people* are to blame if my apartment/house is not a place where I can enjoy life.	1.45	0.82	1-5
External control: Chance:			
3. Having a nice place is all *luck.* You cannot influence it; you just have to accept it.	2.19	1.19	1-5
6. It is purely a matter of *luck* whether or not my neighbors help in an emergency or not.	2.54	1.13	1-5
9. Whether or not I can stay in my apartment/house depends on *fortunate circumstance.*	2.39	1.28	1-5
12. You just have to live with the way your apartment/house is; you *cannot do anything about it.*	1.89	1.11	1-5
15. *Chance* has pretty much determined where and how I live.	2.18	1.27	1-5
18. It is a matter of *luck* whether or not I will be able to pursue my current manner of living in this apartment/house in the future.	2.35	1.21	1-5
21. The way my apartment/house has been set up is something that has more or less *occurred on its own over the years.*	2.34	1.12	1-5
24. Whether or not there are support services or community facilities in my neighborhood is a matter of *luck.*	2.53	1.14	1-5

Note. Items were presented on a five-point rating scale from 1 = "not at all" to 5 = "very much."

of this pilot version of the HCQ particularly with respect to the ECPO dimension was also supported by factor analytic techniques.

Relation of the HCQ with Socio-Structural, General Control Beliefs, and Environment-Related Variables

Housing-related control beliefs and socio-structural variables. The literature on general and domain-specific control beliefs suggests that External Control, but not Internal Control, should be higher in older adults (Lachman, Ziff, & Spiro,1994). Correlating the three housing-related control belief scales with age within Sample B resulted, as expected, in a nonsignificant IC-by-age relation ($r = .08$, n.s.). In contrast, and in accordance with our expectations, both External Control subscales were positively related to age (ECPO: $r = .22$; $p < .05$; ECC: $r = .29$; $p < .01$). This tendency was also confirmed on the mean level by contrasting both samples. Means amounted in the "young-old" Sample A to IC: 3.93 ($SD = .55$), ECPO: 1.88 ($SD = .51$) and ECC: 2.31 ($SD = .79$), while means in Sample B were IC: 4.09 ($SD = .65$), ECPO: 1.86 ($SD = .62$), and ECC: 2.71 ($SD = .87$). In particular, the mean score for ECC tended to be higher in the older sample.

Based on data from the larger sample A, and as expected, gender did not show a relation with Internal Control ($r = .01$, n.s.) and External Control: Powerful Others ($r = -.04$), but a significant, albeit low correlation with External Control: Chance ($r = .13$, $p < .01$). Significant but also rather low correlations were observed with education and household income. In particular, and as might be expected, persons with higher degrees in education and with higher income tended to be lower in both external control subscales.

Housing-related control beliefs and general control beliefs. Correlations in the intermediate range between general control beliefs and domain-specific control beliefs were expected. This was based on assumptions that: (a) housing-specific control beliefs are part of the repertoire of the general control beliefs of individuals; and (b) to the degree the HCQ is tapping into variance unique to the housing domain, both domain-specific and general control beliefs should be unrelated. Assessing the correlations between the three domain-specific scales with the comparable scales of the general control belief questionnaire (Sample A) show a low to intermediate positive correlation between both internal scales, while the relation between the ECPO scales was tentatively negative or nonsubstantial (see Table 2). In contrast, correlations between both HCQ external scales and the general external scales were clearly higher (but never reached more than about 25% of common variance), while the relation with the general internal scales was negative or non-substantial. Thus, the HCQ revealed the expected correlative patterns with a general con-

TABLE 2. Correlation of Housing-Related Control Beliefs Questionnaire Subscales and General Control Beliefs Subscales

Housing-Related Control Beliefs Questionnaire (HCQ)	General Control Beliefs Questionnaire [a]		
	Internal control (subscale)	External control: Powerful others (subscale)	External control: Chance (subscale)
Internal control (subscale)	.27**	−.13**	.05
External control: Powerful others (subscale)	−.07	.38**	.39**
External control: Chance (subscale)	−.14**	.30**	.54**

Note. N = 485 participants from Interdisciplinary Longitudinal Study on Adult Development (ILSE); **p < .01.
[a] Adapted from the Berlin Aging Study (BASE) (Smith, Marsiske, & Maier, 1996; Baltes, Freund, & Horgas, 1999).

trol measure, but these correlations were not so high as to question the need to differentiate between both constructs.

Housing-related control beliefs and environment-related variables. For the present analysis, we selected only those housing-related characteristics expected to be particularly relevant to either internal or external housing-related control beliefs. For instance, with respect to objective environmental aspects, we assumed that owners have more say over their everyday home environments than tenants; subsequently, one would expect their perceptions of internal control to be higher and their perceptions of external control to be lower. Also, the assumption was that more positive aspects, like barrier-free amenities in the objective housing environment or more available space should tentatively come with higher internal and lower external scores in the HCQ, although potential causal dynamics behind such correlations were not considerable (i.e., whether better objective feature impact on housing-related control beliefs or whether housing-related control beliefs impact on the adaptation and improvement of the home environment). In addition, we hypothesized with respect to subjective environmental perceptions that internal housing-related control is positively and external control is negatively related to positive evaluations of the home environment (e.g., perceived housing problems, satisfaction with housing, place attachment, but also the perceived neighborhood safety). Finally, the expectation was that the HCQ should consistently reveal higher correlations with environment-related variables as compared to the general control measure.

As can be seen in Table 3, tenants revealed higher External Control (both subscales) than owners, but this was not the case in terms of higher internal control. Results with respect to other objective features of the home environment confirmed the expected correlative pattern, but on a quite low level of relationship. With regard to perceived housing problems, there was a meaningful negative relationship between lower perceived quality of the home environment and higher Internal Control and a positive relation with both external scales, respectively. Also, both general housing satisfaction and place attachment as well as perceived neighborhood safety were positively related to Internal Control and negatively to both subscores of External Control. Again, however, all of these relations were quite low, but tended to be consistently higher as compared to the general control measure.

DISCUSSION

This work started with the premise that both from the perspective of lifespan development as well as environmental gerontology housing-related con-

TABLE 3. Correlation of Housing-Related versus General Control Beliefs Subscales and Housing Environment-Related Variables

	Housing-Related Control Beliefs Questionnaire (HCQ)			General Control Beliefs Questionnaire[a]		
	Internal control	External control: Powerful others	External control: Chance	Internal control	External control: Powerful others	External control: Chance
Objective housing-related criterion						
Housing tenure (tenant = 0, owner = 1)	.04	−.25**	−.19**	−.06	−.00	−.03
Amount of space (m^2)	.02	−.21**	−.19**	−.04	.01	−.12**
Barrier-free amenities at home (sum score 0-9)	.15**	−.18**	−.08	.05	−.08	−.00
Lighting at home (sum score 0-5)	.19**	−.16**	−.04	.05	−.13**	.02
Objective quality of home (rating 1-5)	.16**	−.21**	−.19	−.03	−.01	−.04
Subjective housing-related criterion						
Perceived housing problems (rating 1-5)	−.16**	.24**	.18**	−.06	.02	.03
Satisfaction with housing (rating 1-5)	.24**	−.29**	−.23**	.06	−.03	−.06
Place attachment to the home environment (rating 1-5)	.22**	−.19**	−.18**	.06	−.11*	−.09*
Perceived neighborhood safety (rating 1-4)	.16**	−.18**	−.11**	.09*	−.05	−.06

Note. N = 485 participants from the Interdisciplinary Longitudinal Study on Adult Development (ILSE). *p < .05; **p < .01. See, for further description of housing environment-related variables, the method section of this work.
[a] Adapted from the Berlin Aging Study (BASE) (Smith, Marsiske, & Maier, 1996; Baltes, Freund, & Horgas, 1999).

trol beliefs should become increasingly important as people age. Housing-related control beliefs were also seen as tapping an important component of what Lawton (1989a) has labeled environmental proactivity, that is, the agency of older persons in terms of arranging their housing situation in accordance with their aging needs and goals. Thus, our first goal was to create a pilot version of an instrument to measure housing-related control beliefs, the Housing-Related Control Beliefs Questionnaire (HCQ), and to examine its psychometric properties. Our second goal was to explore the relation between the HCQ and socio-structural variables, general control beliefs and housing environment-related aspects.

Concerning our first goal, the items of the HCQ were designed to target three theoretically expected dimensions of control, namely Internal Control (IC), External Control: Powerful Others (ECPO), and External Control: Chance (ECC), and a variety of functions of the home environment as suggested in the literature (Lawton, 1989b; Wahl, 2001). Sample A, consisting of 485 old adults, revealed satisfactory internal consistencies comparable to those of Sample B, consisting of 107 old adults. In addition, retest reliability coefficients demonstrated satisfactory stability of the HCQ and factor analysis suggested the expected three-factor solution, explaining a considerable amount of variance with highest loadings of most items on the hypothesized factors.

With regard to the second goal of our study, results from Sample B revealed age correlations in accordance with our theoretical assumptions, i.e., both External Control subscales were positively related to age, whereas Internal Control was not. That is, housing-related control beliefs seem to behave in their age-related variation similar to those concerned with other life domains such as health or intellectual control (e.g., Clark-Plaskie & Lachman, 1999; Lachman, & Weaver, 1998; Lachman, Ziff, & Spiro, 1994). As was also expected, the relation with gender was generally weak, but both higher education and income were related to lower external housing-related control beliefs. Examination of the relationship between the domain-specific measure of housing-related control beliefs and general control beliefs revealed intermediate correlations, suggesting both that housing-specific control beliefs are part of the repertoire of the general control beliefs of individuals, yet the domain-specific HCQ also measures a considerable amount of unique variance. This result supports the interpretation that housing is not only an important part of everyday life in old age (Baltes, Maas, Wilms, Borchelt, & Little, 1999), but a life domain that covers unique experiences and self-regulative processes, including environmental proactivity (Carp & Carp, 1984; Golant, 1998; Lawton, 1989a, 1999; Rubinstein & Parmelee, 1992; Slangen-de Kort, 1999).

Finally, the relation of the HCQ scales with a set of housing-related variables was explored. As expected, housing-related External Control was lower among owners compared to tenants, but the expected higher amount of Internal Control of home owners was not observed. Furthermore, the expectation of lower External Control as well as higher Internal Control among those participants who considered their homes better in terms of objective and subjective indicators was quite consistently confirmed, but all correlations were low in size. They were, however, higher as compared to the correlations of the general control belief measure with housing environment variables.

Although we regard these first results in terms of psychometric quality and content as promising, the real test of the HCQ still is ahead. In particular, we will examine the predictive validity of the instrument in a heterogeneous sample, which was not available in the present study, in which both samples were positively biased due to their age (Sample A, only young-old participants) or recruitment strategy (Sample B, generated via newspaper announcements). An additional disadvantage of the present study was that data-collection took place not in the home environment of the participants, but in a "laboratory" setting. That is, all environment-related variables were assessed based on participants' reports and not on a real observation/assessment of their housing situation. To counteract these limitations of the current work, a new project entitled "Enable Age" (Oswald, Wahl, & Mollenkopf, 2001) is underway. This project will focus on a detailed description of the home environment of a random sample of very old persons (Iwarsson & Slaug, 2001) and will use the HCQ as a means to predict emotional and behavioral outcomes across a one-year interval. Our hypothesis is that very old individuals high in housing-related Internal Control should have a stronger tendency towards actively optimizing their home environment and to create for themselves an "enabling" environment (Steinfeld & Danford, 1999; see also Lanspery & Hyde, 1997), as compared to those higher in housing-related External Control. If these hypotheses find empirical support, then the HCQ may serve as a potential tool to inform and support practical and intervention decisions concerned with housing older adults in the future.

REFERENCES

Abeles, R. P. (1991). Sense of control, quality of life, and frail older people. In J. E. Birren, D. E. Deutschmann, J. Lubben & J. Rowe (Eds.), *The concept of measurement of quality of life in the frail elderly* (pp. 297-314). New York: Academic Press.

Baltes, P. B., & Baltes, M. M. (Eds.). (1986). *The psychology of control and aging.* Hillsdale, NJ: Lawrence Erlbaum.

Baltes, M. M., Freund, A. M., & Horgas, A. L. (1999). Men and women in the Berlin Aging Study. In P. B. Baltes & K. U. Mayer (Eds.), *The Berlin Aging Study* (pp. 259-281). Cambridge: Cambridge University Press.

Baltes, M. M., Maas, I., Wilms, H.-U., Borchelt, M., & Little, T. D. (1999). Everyday competence in old and very old age: Theoretical considerations and empirical findings. In P. B. Baltes & K. U. Mayer (Eds.), *The Berlin Aging Study* (pp. 384-402). Cambridge: Cambridge University Press.

Bandura, A. (Ed.). (1995). *Self-efficacy in changing societies.* New York: Cambridge University Press.

Brandstädter, J., & Renner, G. (1990). Tenacious goal pursuit and flexible goal adjustment: Explication and age-related analysis of assimilative and accommodative strategies of coping. *Psychology and Aging, 5*, 58-67.

Carp, F. M., & Carp, A. (1984). A complementary/congruence model of well-being or mental health for the community elderly. In I. Altman, M. P. Lawton & J. F. Wohlwill (Eds.), *Human behavior and environment: Vol. 7. Elderly people and the environment* (pp. 279-336). New York: Plenum Press.

Clark-Plaskie, M., & Lachman, M. E. (1999). The sense of control in midlife. In S. L. Willis & J. D. Reid (Eds.), *Life in the middle: Psychological and social development in middle age* (pp. 181-208). San Diego, CA: Academic Press.

Golant, S. M. (1998). Changing an older person's shelter and care setting: A model to explain personal and environmental outcomes. In R. J. Scheidt & P. G. Windley (Eds.), *Environment and aging theory. A focus on housing* (pp. 33-60). Westport, CT: Greenwod Press.

Havighurst, R. J. (1972). *Developmental tasks and education* (3rd ed.). New York: McKay.

Iwarsson, S., & Slaug, B. (2001). *Housing Enabler. An instrument for assessing and analyzing accessibility problems in housing.* Lund (Sweden): Studentlitteratur.

Lachman, M. E. (1986). Locus of control in aging research: A case for multidimensional and domain-specific assessment. *Journal of Psychology and Aging, 1*, 34-40.

Lachman, M. E. (Ed.). (1993). Planning and control processes across the life span: An overview [Special issue]. *International Journal of Behavioral Development, 16.*

Lachman, M. E., & Weaver, S. L. (1998). Sociodemographic variations in the sense of control by domain: Findings from the MacArthur studies of midlife. *Psychology and Aging, 13*, 553-562.

Lachman, M. E., Ziff, M., & Spiro, A. (1994). Maintaining a sense of control in later life. In R. P. Abeles, H. C. Gift, & M. G. Ory (Eds.), *Aging and quality of life* (pp. 216-232). New York: Springer Publishing Co.

Lanspery, S., & Hyde, J. (Eds.). (1997). *Staying put. Adapting the places instead of the people.* Amityville, NY: Baywood.

Lawton, M. P. (1983). Environment and other determinants of well-being in older people. *The Gerontologist, 23*(4), 349-357.

Lawton, M. P. (1985). Housing and living environments of older people. In R. H. Binstock & E. Shanas (Eds.), *Handbook of Aging and the Social Sciences* (2nd ed., pp. 450-478). New York: Van Nostrand Reinhold.

Lawton, M. P. (1987). Environment and the need satisfaction of the aging. In L. L. Carstensen & B. A. Edelstein (Eds.), *Handbook of clinical gerontology* (pp. 33-40). New York: Pergamon Press.

Lawton, M. P. (1989a). Environmental Proactivity in Older People. In V.L. Bengtson & K. W. Schaie (Eds.), *The Course of Later Life* (pp. 15-23). New York: Springer.

Lawton, M. P. (1989b). Three functions of the residential environment. In L. A. Pastalan & M. E. Cowart (Eds.), *Lifestyle and housing of older adults: The Florida experience* (pp. 35-50). New York: The Haworth Press, Inc.

Lawton, M. P. (1998). Environment and aging: Theory revisited. In R. J. Scheidt & P. G. Windley (Eds.), *Environment and aging theory. A focus on housing* (pp. 1-32). Westport: Greenwood Press.

Lawton, M. P. (1999). Environmental taxonomy: Generalizations from research with older adults. In S. L. Friedman & T. D. Wachs (Eds.), *Measuring environment across the life span* (pp. 91-124). Washington, DC: American Psychological Association.

Levenson, H. (1973). Multidimensional locus of control in psychiatric patients. *Journal of Consulting and Clinical Psychology*, 41, 397-404.

Levenson, H. (1981). Differentiating among internality, powerful others, and chance. In H. M. Lefcourt (Ed.), *Research with the locus of control construct: Vol 1. Assessment methods*. New York: Academic Press.

Martin, P., Ettrich, K. U., Lehr, U., Roether, D., Martin, M., & Fischer-Cyrulies, A. (Eds.). (2000). *Aspekte der Entwicklung im mittleren und höheren Lebensalters. Ergebnisse der Interdisziplinären Längsschnittstudie des Erwachsenenalters (ILSE). [Developmental aspects in middle and late adulthood. Results from the Interdisciplinary Longitudinal Study on Adult Development (ILSE).]* Darmstadt: Steinkopff.

Moen, P., & Wethington, E. (1999). Midlife development in a life course context. In S. L. Willis & J. D. Reid (Eds.), *Life in the middle: Psychological and social development in middle age* (pp. 3-23). San Diego, CA: Academic Press.

Moss, M. S., & Lawton, M. P. (1982). Time budgets of older people: A window of four lifestyles. *Journal of Gerontology*, 37, 115-123.

Oswald, F., Wahl, H.-W., & Mollenkopf, H. (2001). *Enhancing autonomy and health-related abilities in old age: The role of the home environment* (ENABLE-AGE). Project funded by the European Commission (in conjunction with partners from England, Hungary, Latvia, and Sweden).

Parmelee, P. A., & Lawton, M. P. (1990). The design of special environments for the aged. In J. E. Birren & K. W. Schaie (Eds.), *Handbook of the psychology of aging* (3rd ed., pp. 464-488). New York: Academic Press.

Pynoos, J. (1995). Home modifications. In G. L. Maddox (Ed.), *The encyclopedia of aging. A comprehensive resource in gerontology and geriatrics* (2nd ed., pp. 466-469). New York: Springer.

Reich, J. W., & Zautra, A. J. (1990). Dispositional control beliefs and the consequences of a control-enhancing intervention. *Journal of Gerontology: Psychological Sciences*, 45, P46-51.

Rubinstein, R. L., & Parmelee, P. A. (1992). Attachment to place and the representation of life course by the elderly. In I. Altman & S. M. Low (Eds.), *Human behavior and environment: Vol. 12. Place Attachment* (pp. 139-163). New York: Plenum Press.

Schaie, K. W., Wahl, H.-W., Mollenkopf, H., & Oswald, F. (Eds.). (in press). *Aging in the community: Living arrangements and mobility*. New York: Springer Publishing Co.

Scheidt, R. J. (1998). The social ecology approach of Rudolf Moos. In R. J. Scheidt & P. G. Windley (Eds.), *Environment and aging theory. A focus on housing* (pp. 111-139). Westport, CT: Greenwod Press.

Schulz, R., & Brenner, G. (1977). Relocation of the aged: A review and theoretical analysis. *Journal of Gerontology, 32,* 323-333.

Schulz, R., & Heckhausen, J. (1997). Emotions and control: A life span perspective. In M. P. Lawton & K. W. Schaie (Eds.), *Annual review of gerontology and geriatrics* (Vol. 17, pp. 185-205). New York: Springer Publishing Co.

Schulz, R., & Heckhausen, J. (1999). Aging, culture and control: Setting a new research agenda. *Journal of Gerontology: Psychological Sciences, 54B,* P139-145.

Seligman, M. E. P. (1991). *Learned optimism.* New York: Knopf.

Skinner, E. A. (1995). *Perceived control, motivation, and coping.* Thousand Oaks, CA: Sage.

Slangen-de Kort, Y. A. W. (1999). *A tale of two adaptations.* Eindhoven University of Technology: University Press.

Slangen-de Kort, Y. A. W., Midden, C. J. H., & Wagenberg, A. F. (1998). Predictors of the adaptive problem solving of older persons in their homes. *Journal of Environmental Psychology, 18,* 187-197.

Smith, J., Marsiske, M., & Maier, H. (1996). *Differences in control beliefs from age 70 to 105.* Unpublished manuscript. Max Planck Institute for Human Development, Berlin.

Steinfeld, E., & Danford, G. S. (Eds.). (1999). *Enabling environments. Measuring the impact of environment on disability and rehabilitation.* New York: Plenum Press.

Timko, C., & Moss, R. H. (1989). Choice, control, and adaptation among elderly residents of sheltered care settings. *Journal of Applied Social Psychology, 19,* 636-655.

Wahl, H.-W. (2001). Environmental influences on aging and behavior. In J. E. Birren & K. W. Schaie (Eds.), *Handbook of the psychology of aging* (5th ed., pp. 215-237). San Diego, CA: Academic Press.

Index

T - #0571 - 101024 - C0 - 212/152/9 - PB - 9780789020079 - Gloss Lamination